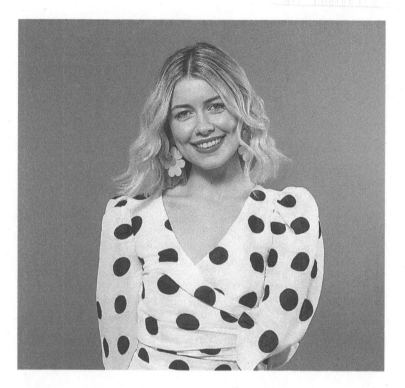

Bridget Hustwaite is the Melbourne-based host of triple j's flagship new music program Good Nights. A trusted and respected voice in the music industry, Bridget also uses her platform to raise awareness for endometriosis, a condition with which she was diagnosed in 2018. Following the outpouring of support she received for sharing her story on triple j, Bridget launched the Instagram account @endogram, which aims to educate and start conversations about endometriosis with its 20K+ followers.

how

to

a guide to
surviving and
thriving with
endometriosis

endo

bridget hustwaite

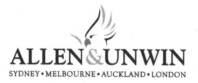

ALLEN&UNWIN
SYDNEY · MELBOURNE · AUCKLAND · LONDON

First published in 2021

Allen & Unwin
83 Alexander Street
Crows Nest NSW 2065
Australia
Phone: (61 2) 8425 0100
Email: info@allenandunwin.com
Web: www.allenandunwin.com

A catalogue record for this book is available from the National Library of Australia

ISBN 978 1 76087 908 2

Internal design by Alissa Dinallo
Internal illustrations by Mika Tabata
Index by Kerryn Burgess
Set in 11/16 pt Filson Pro Book by Bookhouse, Sydney
Printed and bound in Australia by the Opus Group

10 9 8 7

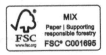

MIX
Paper | Supporting
responsible forestry
FSC® C001695

For fifteen-year-old Bridget,
who knew her shitty periods
weren't normal

Contents

HOW TO HELP — 229

Welcome!

I'll be honest: I have NO idea how to start this thing! Which may seem strange for someone who can confidently greet a national audience on live radio every single weeknight. But this is very different.

Much like with writing, there is a structure when it comes to radio presenting. Even though there are a lot of announcers out there who have this wonderful ability to sound quite spontaneous and casual, we've all been trained to follow *some* kind of formula. For instance, the first talk break of my show is the most important one to nail because it will basically determine whether or not the listener will stay tuned or switch stations. The general flow is this:

Greeting (Hi! What's up! Welcome!) > Forward Promote (Here's what's coming up/why you need to stay tuned) > Play First Song.

All in all, it takes about 90 seconds. Usually with some audio grabs to keep it colourful but it needs to be straight to the point. Keep it tight and adapt a 'word economy', as my former boss would call it.

It is the absolute opposite of writing a book, where there is simply no such thing. Instead, you are punching towards *tens of thousands* of words. Allllll the words. I'm freeeeee to say as much as I want!

So, hi! It's nice to meet you and I'm so excited that you have picked up this book. You may have done so because:

- You're searching for an endometriosis diagnosis
- You have already been diagnosed
- You have a loved one with endometriosis and you want to learn more about it
- None of the above—maybe you listen to me on the radio or thought this book looked cool (don't blame you). ¯_(ツ)_/¯

Whatever the reason, I'm glad you're here and I want you to know a few things before you dive in. Like why I have decided to write a book on endometriosis. Well, you could say that experiencing the blows of this chronic illness firsthand has sparked a real fire in my belly. I mean, she was already inflamed but I just don't want others to deal with what I had to. The physical damage, the emotional distress, the constant dismissal. Not to mention all the things I was never told or warned about when it came to navigating life with an incurable disease with no known cause. My journey of personal research and self-advocacy has been long and confusing. I mean, where do you even start? *How do you endo?*

In a perfect world, this book wouldn't even need to exist because there would be sufficient awareness, research and funding surrounding endometriosis. You'd be taken seriously by doctors and have access to the right treatments. Your loved ones would understand and your relationships would continue to blossom. You would feel supported in your professional life and personal ambitions, whatever they may be.

Alas, this perfect world is not yet ready for us so, in the meantime, let this book be a way to comfort you through the shitty times and to reassure you that what you are feeling is very real. Let it educate you on the things that so many of us were never taught. Hopefully, it saves you some coin as well, because managing endo ain't always cheap.

But I hope some of my personal advice, as well as the expertise of others, will help you make informed choices that are friendly to your body and your wallet. I'm certainly no medical professional and while I don't have all the answers, I hope this book is enough to get you going on the right path. Think of this book as a set of training wheels while you learn to ride a bike. We might be a bit wobbly sometimes but ideally by the end, you'll be ready to pedal off into the sunset on your own. Just remember which side the front brake is on so you're not sent flying over the handlebars, okay?

Nobody likes a spoiler, but it is important that you know that there is no single way to live with this disease. There is no standard fit to surviving and thriving with endo because, just like adulting, we are still figuring it out. Plus, everybody's end goal is different, but that doesn't mean you are alone in this journey. Let this book be a way of us doing it together.

So, you ready?

Let's get into it!

"Tell the story of the mountains you climbed. Your words could become a page in someone else's survival guide."

MORGAN HARPER NICHOLS

My story

'OMG, I think this is my period?!'

Ahhh, your first time. Hard to forget, isn't it? Mine was during the first week of Year 7 which made for a timely welcome to high school. I remember power walking (read: smugly strutting) to the toilets with a liner hidden in my dress pocket, giggling as my new friends followed in excitement. I was one of the first in my friendship group to receive a visit from Aunty Flow. I mean, it wasn't a competition, but this new experience made me feel pretty cool (or kewl, cos 2003). Plus, Mum had said she would buy me a new teddy bear when I got it and as an eleven-year-old going on twelve, I still very much loved my plush toys. I didn't think too much into *why* Mum felt like I needed a new bear, or 'period bear' as she emphasised. I was just pumped to add a new one to the collection sitting cosily on my bed.

The first few cycles were fine, just some light bleeding that only required liners. But soon enough, I came to understand the purpose of Poppy the Pink Period Bear. You see, instead of a gradual increase in flow, duration and general discomfort, my period decided to go from zero to 100. Like, it was a real nek-minute situation. Those first period giggles were quickly replaced with groans, while that smug strut to the toilet became more of a walk of shame. I was popping more painkillers than any normal menstruating teen should require and awkwardly asking Mum to buy me overnight pads because 'regular' just didn't cut it. I found myself wearing multiple pairs of undies to prevent leaking and the only way to wear my school jumper during shark week was tied around my waist. Even if the weather suggested otherwise, I was willing to risk the cold for no red marks. Come summertime, the most commonly asked question you'd get from me was never regarding curriculum. It was instead to my friends as we got up at the end of each class: 'Can you check the back of my dress?'

Poppy was a much-needed comfort because my period was just as inconvenient at home. I avoided using the nice, fluffy towels after a shower in case I ruined them with stains. I would sleep on an old towel to prevent the blood from leaking on to my sheets. I even remember blood literally pouring out of my vagina and straight on to the carpet one morning in my bedroom, as I'd been too slow in changing my underwear and pad. By the way, there is no such thing as too much information in this book. The sooner we normalise period conversations, the better, because I know I'm not the only one who has dealt with this! Anyway, I was horrified by what had happened and scared that I would get in trouble for the stain. I can still hear the concern in my mum's voice:

'You always have bad periods.' Up until this point, I thought that maybe everybody dealt with such bullshit cycles and they were just better at hiding it. But my two sisters never had periods like mine, and Mum's concern was enough to suggest that we should do something.

I first saw a doctor about my period in Year 10, so I would have been fifteen at the time. Endometriosis was not in my vocabulary and I guess it wasn't in the doctor's either. I was prescribed Levlen, a contraceptive pill, and sent on my way. To say I hated taking the Pill would be an understatement. I know birth control works differently for everyone but, for me, the pill triggered weight gain and I still experienced the physical symptoms of my period. It would start with a pulsing headache, which I learned to recognise as my body's way of saying, 'Heads up, Aunty Flow's coming to visit and she isn't happy.' And the cramps, UGH the cramps! I flinch whenever I think of those dull, nauseating throbs that felt like my ovaries were in a punch-on before they were doused in petrol and set on fire.

Then came sex. I lost my virginity to my first serious boyfriend when I was eighteen. I expected it to hurt because, you know, I was new to the whole thing, but the pain just didn't feel right. It felt like it was more than just typical cherry-poppin' pain and it continued for a long time. Throughout our relationship, it was common for us to have to stop mid-sex because the sharp, burning sensation would just take over. I would then crawl into the foetal position and wonder, *What is wrong with me?* I remember it being so bad one night that I just got up and drove back home because the best way to suffer was in the comfort of my own bed. My first boyfriend never made me feel like it was my fault, but I knew that he knew it wasn't normal. After our relationship ended, my sexual encounters were rare and usually involved alcohol. Looking back on it now, I feel like the alcohol was a way of masking how my body was really feeling.

Three years out of high school and the pain extended to my abdominal area. I was two weeks into my Visual Merchandising diploma in Melbourne, when I suddenly experienced a sharp, stabbing sensation along my belly one afternoon during class. It was such an unfamiliar feeling and, at the time, I thought it was the result of something I'd eaten. I sat there, squirming in my seat and gripping the edge of the table until I could take no more and stumbled out of the classroom, hunched over. I was taken to the ER in an ambulance, asked if I was pregnant and received strong pain relief until I felt better. Nurses and doctors didn't do tests or scans, and I didn't know what to ask for. Endometriosis still didn't exist to me, let alone the knowledge that this was a likely symptom.

For the following four years, this pain would strike at any given moment. Like during a retail shift when I was running the store by myself and had to wait nearly two hours for my regional manager to come and take over. Or at dinner in Korčula in Croatia with my friends, where I had no choice but to get up and run back to my cabin before the food arrived. I still mourn that Margherita pizza, RIP. Even on one of my first dates with my current partner, he genuinely wasn't sure if I was in pain or just making it up to get out of the date—we'd paid, like, $40 to ice skate and I hate wasting money so rest assured, Jenno, I wasn't faking it!

In 2015, I was referred for an endoscopy. The only conclusion my doctor made from that procedure was the potential risk of high acid levels in my stomach—but nothing definitive. While this random abdominal pain was plotting its next attack on my body, things were Absolutely Not Improving on the period front. I could sense its impending arrival in the form of extreme cravings for chocolate, followed by a throbbing, nauseating pain and then a nice blood clot or two sitting in my undies, as if to say, 'I'm baaack and bearing gifts!' My cycle got shorter and shorter; my period returned every three weeks, sometimes fortnightly. The pain on the first day would knock me so hard I would often have to call in sick to work. I felt heavy, sluggish, pretty darn useless and had no choice but to start scheduling my life around my period.

Throughout this time, I sought advice from numerous GPs. Only one took my case seriously enough to provide a referral for a gynaecologist but I was earning peanuts as a travel agent and simply could not afford the consultation fee. It was literally a choice of either paying for groceries that week or having the appointment, so you can guess which one I went with. I think this GP may have been the first professional to mention the word endometriosis, but it was mainly through my friend Hayleigh that I grasped a rough idea of what this condition entailed. We worked in retail together before I become a travel agent, and I remember her having to take days off before receiving her diagnosis. But we never got too deep into the discussion and I can't help but think it was due to us feeling silenced by the menstrual taboo.

In 2017, I was back living at home with my parents in Ballarat and had some money saved, so I decided to see a local female GP who was recommended to me based on her specialisation in women's health. Alongside a gynaecologist referral, I also needed a pap smear and something for a cold I had, so I made sure to call up in advance and book a longer appointment. I was beyond excited at the thought of seeing someone who would finally understand my pain, but it turned out to be my most disappointing encounter with a medical professional. Ever. From the moment I entered the room, this GP didn't want a bar of me. I'm not sure if she was having a bad day but the whole time, she was beyond disinterested. Closed body language, no eye contact. It looked like it took every last ounce of strength for her not to eyeroll. And then she said it. 'You don't have endometriosis. Others have it worse than you.'

Talk about a shutdown! You know that scene from *The Simpsons* where Lisa tells Ralph she never liked him and Bart replays it to her? 'You can actually pinpoint the second when his heart rips in half!' It kinda felt like that.

I didn't know the diagnostic process for endo but this felt Very Off, so I persisted for a gynae referral. 'I'll give you one, but I don't think you need it,' she sighed as she handed me the letter. As for the cold, I got an antibiotics prescription. The pap smear? 'We can do it next time.' Umm? What about my extended appointment? But, honestly, I was so shook by this entire consult that I just walked out, returned to my car and sat wondering what the fuck just happened. I didn't follow through with the gynaecologist, again, but it wasn't about money this time around. I actually feared that the GP was going to call up the gynaecologist and warn them about me or something.

After moving to Sydney for my dream job in 2018 and securing a good, stable income, I thought it was the perfect chance to have another crack. I needed to get on top of my pain, find a decent GP and follow through with it. A few google searches of 'women's health doctor' led me to a doctor who I found to be so warm, attentive and compassionate as I railed off my history of pain and symptoms.

She had no doubt that it was endometriosis and not only referred me to a gynaecologist but also for an ultrasound straight away. Next thing I knew, I was chugging a litre of water in preparation for this examination, which my sensitive bladder absolutely despised. I had no idea what to expect and since it was my first scan of this kind, I was both curious and nervous. What if it hurt? What if they didn't find anything? What if I peed myself before we even began? Thankfully, the sonographer made the process as comfortable as it could be and while the scan picked up a few cysts on my ovaries, no endometriosis could be detected. I was assured that this was not the be-all and end-all, so I tried not to feel deflated by these findings.

My first appointment with the gynaecologist went well. He was friendly, attentive and after performing an internal examination, he was pretty confident that all signs pointed to endometriosis, despite the ultrasound not picking up any clear indication of the disease. We agreed to do a diagnostic laparoscopy, which basically meant keyhole surgery through my abdomen. But because I didn't have private health insurance, I wasn't going to have this gynaecologist operate on me. Instead, he would be supervising students in training. I wasn't fussed, I was happy to be the guinea pig if it meant no exorbitant out-of-pocket costs. The waitlist for surgery was five months but work was busy, so I didn't have a problem with an August date. Even though it meant enduring five more painful periods and taking various sick days, I was very chill about it all. Had I known the extent of my endometriosis however, I probably would have gone about things differently.

The night before surgery, Jenno arrived from Melbourne. We were navigating a long-distance relationship and, luckily, he'd scored some time off work to fly up to Sydney and look after me for five days. It felt so comforting to have a familiar face there with me but the nerves were hard to shake. I remember crying as we got ready for bed. *What if it's really bad? What if they don't find anything?*

To be honest, I was more terrified of the latter and my pain remaining a mystery. All I wanted was answers and the next day, I got them. Stage four endometriosis. Both superficial and deep infiltrating lesions were found and excised from my bladder, pelvic side walls, distal rectum and pouch of Douglas, which is the small area between the uterus and rectum. I'd also agreed to have an IUD inserted during the procedure as I'd been told it could help manage my pain and 'reduce the likelihood of my endo growing back'. Given my experience with the contraceptive pill, I was really hesitant to try another form of hormonal treatment, but I figured I wouldn't know unless I tried. The surgery took twice as long as expected and due to the extent of my endo, I had to stay overnight.

Waking from anaesthesia has always been hit-and-miss with me. Having gone under eight times before this surgery (for different procedures—knees, ears . . . my body, she is a hot mess!), I have found that my mindset can really affect how I respond to the drug. I remember when I got my tonsils out, I sat up in the recovery ward as soon as I came to and started laughing hysterically because I thought everyone was clapping for me like I was a hero, returning victorious from the war that was tonsillitis and glandular fever. Whereas for my left knee lateral release, I was another kind of hysteric in the form of uncontrollable sobbing. Luckily, I was pretty chill waking from this laparoscopy and based on my first question to the nurse, my procedure was not even front of mind. 'Can we watch the Honey Badger?' It was a *really* good season of *The Bachelor*, okay?

My diagnosis was bittersweet. I was absolutely stoked to hear that there was a reason behind my pain—it felt *so* validating to know it wasn't all in my head or that I was weak. Sure, it sucked that there was no cure, but I didn't ponder that much as I was distracted by all the lovely messages I was receiving. My colleagues at triple j documented my experience for our flagship youth affairs program, *Hack*. Given that triple j is our national youth broadcaster and reaches millions of people, having my story shared on air and across their social media platforms really blew up my inbox. I received *hundreds and hundreds* of messages from our listeners—who were all reaching out for various reasons. Some had already been diagnosed, some were seeking answers and others had someone in their life going through the same thing. Hearing how my experience helped other people learn about endo or have those important conversations with their loved ones brought me so much comfort in my recovery. Even through the aching of my abdomen and the intense shoulder tip pressure from the gas used to allow better viewing of my organs, I was feeling confident that I could bounce back from this. I even emailed the GP from Ballarat to share my diagnosis and the links to the online coverage surrounding it. I wasn't expecting a response, nor did I receive one, but it felt good.

Then, reality kicked in. Jenno was due to return home so I would no longer have his warm, comforting hand as he helped me walk, eat, medicate, shower and pee (he really saw it all). I don't know how I could have done those first few days without him and was devastated when he left. I was still struggling with my new life in Sydney and the thought of having to combat the rest of my recovery alone was terrifying. The process was harder and slower than I anticipated, and it really took all my strength. It took twice as long to get ready for work and I would sit with a heat pack right until I had to leave. The train station was too far away for me to walk to in my sore state, as was the bus stop, so for six weeks I took a rideshare to work. In the evening, I would return home absolutely exhausted and with the dread of having to do it all again the next day. I often found myself softly sobbing in my room, completely overwhelmed and alone in my thoughts. I was living in a four-bedroom share house with people I rarely saw due to our differing work schedules, and while I know they would have helped if I had asked, I always insisted I was fine. In my stubbornness to be independent and my fear of losing control, I would also downplay my pain to my colleagues and friends. It felt more convenient than trying to explain what my recovery really entailed and, looking back now, this turned out to be a pretty toxic way of internalising my suffering, because I saw it as my body and therefore my problem.

I thought that once the endo was removed, the pain would disappear. My gynaecologist said that the IUD could take up to six months for my body to adjust to and, naturally, I trusted him.

But my body wasn't the same. I bled for weeks following surgery, which I think was due to a combination of recovery and my period deciding to rear its ugly head. Instead of being able to exercise after six weeks as I was told, it took five months to do it pain-free. Five. Months. One of the harshest realisations I had of the long road ahead was ten days following the surgery, when I attempted a slow, solo walk to a local BONDS outlet, a one-kilometre stroll from home. I was determined to stock up on some comfortable trackies and even more determined to make the distance on foot. Each small step was met with discomfort, but it wasn't until the final 100 metres that an overwhelming sensation washed painfully across my pelvic area like a crashing wave, making me really light-headed. I could feel my vision fading as the giant cramp within my cervix intensified, like my IUD was banging the walls, trying to escape. I crouched down on the pavement and tried to call one of my housemates in the hope that she could pick me up, but she didn't answer. I eventually mustered the strength to hobble the last hundred metres—did I mention I'm pretty stubborn? I mean, I could see the store ahead. I was so close! *Nothing* was going to come between me and these trackies, but you bet I ordered a rideshare home. I remember sinking into the back seat with my purchase, completely exhausted and astounded at how an innocent walk to the shop could turn into such a gruelling ordeal, with the driver completely unaware as we made the one-kilometre trip home.

Sex was still painful and I began to experience random flare-ups that felt like a sharp, burning pressure, unlike anything I had dealt with before. It would strike at any given time—on a plane, in the car, riding a bike, lying in bed, you name it. I felt stalked by my own body (or my own pain) and, as a result, I developed a lot of anxiety. I was scared to socialise or be anywhere without my heat pack. It felt safer to isolate and while I remained chirpy on air during my radio show, I was turning into a shell outside of work.

I couldn't adjust to life in Sydney so at the end of 2018, I returned to Melbourne and was lucky enough to bring my job back with me. Jenno and I found an apartment to rent together and everything started to feel like it was falling into place. The random flare-ups still struck at their own convenience, but being home was a huge boost to my mental state and I was ready to take on 2019.

At 2 a.m. on the morning of my first day back at work, I suddenly woke in the most excruciating pain. It was a sharp sensation completely overwhelming the lower area of my abdomen. It might sound odd but there are definitely different types of sharp pain and this one was completely foreign to me. I immediately knew that I needed to go to hospital, but I couldn't move. I shrieked in agony, shocking Jenno awake. With one arm over his shoulder, I limped to the car and we drove straight to emergency. I tried to stay calm as I angled my body awkwardly in the passenger seat, but, man, I don't think I have ever dropped so many f-bombs as during that twenty-minute drive.

The pain intensified as we arrived at the emergency room and I was sobbing as I tried to explain what I was feeling while reciting my name and address to the triage nurse. They took me in straight away as they suspected I was pregnant. I definitely wasn't. I was worried they would think I was there just for drugs as I had heard some ER horror stories from other people with endo, but the nurses believed my suffering and kept me in for thirteen hours. I was wheeled to the ultrasound room at 9 a.m., and they confirmed that a haemorrhagic cyst had burst. Haemorr-who? Turns out they're some blood-filled baddies, and a 0/10 experience that I would not recommend. I was also told that my left ovary was immobile. I wasn't entirely sure what that meant but an ovary that was seemingly stuck didn't sound good. I was sent home with a script for Endone and told to come back for a follow-up appointment in eight weeks to see if any more cysts had decided to show up uninvited, like a nosy neighbour. No treatment plan, just a 'see how you go'.

Eight months after my diagnosis, I continued to receive DMs and questions from my followers about my endometriosis. I had no idea just how common this condition was, nor how interested people continued to be in my experience. Because of this, I decided to launch a separate Instagram page dedicated to sharing information and raising awareness. Fittingly named endogram (full credit to Mum), this account led me to undertake a great deal of research and, holy guacamole, I was actually shocked at how little I knew! I didn't realise the extent of this disease at all and what it meant for my life. I didn't even know the importance of excising endo rather than ablating it—which you'll learn all about in Chapter 3. I got lucky with my diagnostic laparoscopy using the preferred removal technique, but I was still experiencing these new flare-ups and I knew that I needed to seek a second opinion.

Because I had returned to Melbourne, I needed to find a new specialist and after consulting a few different local support groups, I found my guy. I put together a manila folder with my full endometriosis history—every scan, my operation notes and photos, my ER admission notes—everything. He examined the photographs from my first laparoscopy and said while they did a good job of excising the disease, he suspected not all of it was correctly removed. This, alongside my recent ultrasounds detecting an immobile left ovary, was enough for him to recommend another surgery.

Noooooooo!

Part of me expected this response but I couldn't help bursting into tears. I was only just starting to feel semi-normal again so the thought of going through another surgery was so draining. I did not feel ready. However, because I had only just taken out private health insurance, I needed to wait ten more months for the waiting period to end, so we booked in for June 2020.

The time leading up to my second surgery was *extremely* weird. COVID-19 had made its way into Victoria and we were in lockdown. Businesses closed, working from home was the new normal for those who could do so and hospitals had no choice but to reduce their theatre capacity. Instead of operating four days a week, my specialist was only operating every Wednesday. A wall of anxiety tumbled over me—*what if my surgery gets delayed? How long will I have to wait? What if there is endometriosis that is worsening? What if it's too late for my immobile left ovary?* It also didn't help that my period decided to show up for three consecutive months and the flare-ups became more frequent. Luckily, my procedure not only went ahead but it was six days earlier than planned, thanks to my private health insurance waiving the three days left on my waiting period.

On 10 June 2020, I had my second excision surgery through the private health system and my specialist's suspicions were confirmed. Severe endometriosis was on my pouch of Douglas and pelvic side walls—not a recurrence, but leftover disease from the first surgery. I also opted, after much consideration, for my IUD to be taken out. The entire procedure took two hours and I stayed two nights in hospital with a drainage tube to remove any extra fluids in my body and a catheter to let my bladder rest. I was super sore and found the removal of the drainage tube to be one of the grossest feelings ever but, despite all this, I had a really good experience. I was lucky to have my own room that had a beautiful view of some of Melbourne's skyline and golden hour was sahhh glorious. All of my nurses were fantastic and my specialist was incredibly diligent. He visited me the night of my surgery with operation notes and photographs but, naturally, I was off my rocker, so I don't remember too much. The next morning, I asked about my IUD, as I was curious to know what state it was in before its removal.

He responded, 'It was sideways.'

Cooooooool, love that for me!

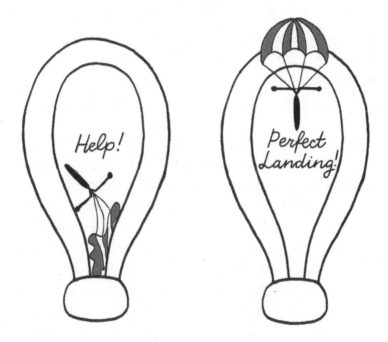

My IUD versus a normal IUD

Recovery this time around was different from my first procedure in many ways. In some respects, it felt better—I didn't have any shoulder tip pain like I'd had previously from the gas used in surgery! On the other hand, I ended up sleeping on our little two-seater couch for the first week because our mattress felt too hard on my tender body. I also needed double the time off work (four weeks as opposed to two) and experienced a mild nerve injury called neuropraxia which felt like some sort of electrical shot throughout my upper thigh, but which thankfully passed. My first two periods after surgery were pretty horrendous, but I am yet to experience a random flare-up, which I can't help but link to having the IUD removed.

It's been a long journey and it's still ongoing because chronic illness, bby. You'll hear more bits from my experience throughout the book but TL;DR:

- too many years dealing with unexplained pain
- too much incorrect info from doctors
- two surgeries
- I'm a boss.

For real though, my endometriosis has taught me so many things. It has taught me to listen to my body because I'm the only true expert of it and I deserve the best care. It has reminded me of my strength and it has helped me find my voice. Which sounds weird given how often people hear me on the radio, but you know what I mean. Ultimately, it's exposed a real drive to share my learnings, my mistakes, everything with other people—those who have been through it, those who are about to but don't know where to start, and anyone who is looking after them.

what to know

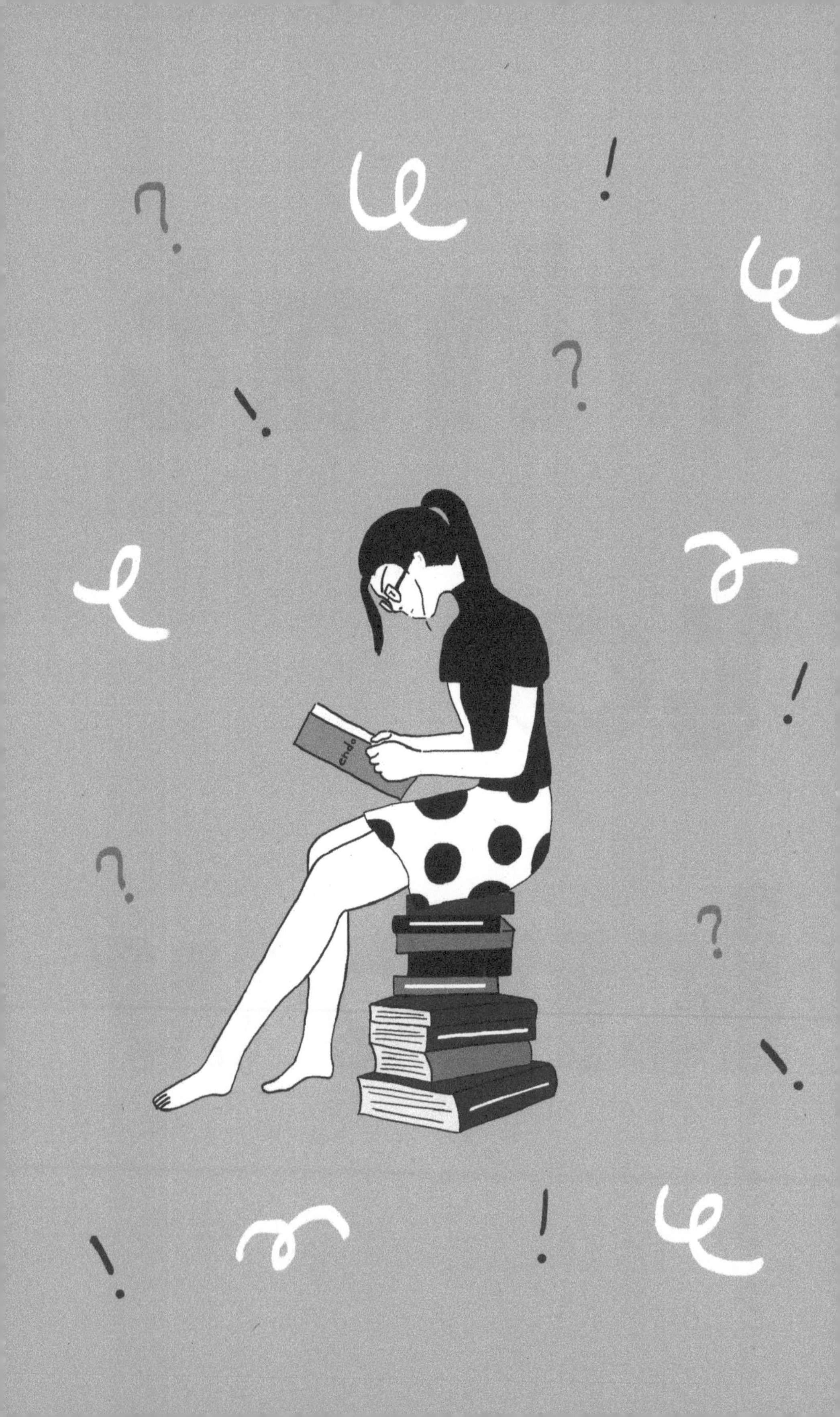
endo

1

Endo 101

Endome . . . *muffled mumbling*
   Close . . .
   Endo . . . metri . . . huh?
   Getting closer . . .
   Endocalifragilisticexpialidocious?
   Okay chill, Mary Poppins. Let's start again.

En-doh-me-tree-oh-sis

So, you've just read about my experience with this painful thing that has a weird name and you're probably wondering, *What the heck is going on down there*? Well, it's complicated but consider this a crash course on the disease that's hard to say, see and solve. Welcome to Endo 101!

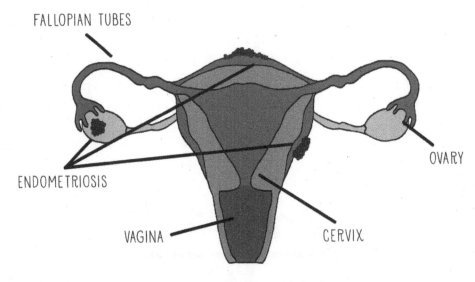

FALLOPIAN TUBES

ENDOMETRIOSIS

VAGINA

OVARY

CERVIX

Diagram of endometriosis

Endometriosis, or endo for short, is a chronic inflammatory condition in which cells that are *similar* to the lining of the uterus (endometrium) grow outside of this layer and result in Pain with a capital P, inflammation, organ dysfunction and, in some cases, infertility. I put an emphasis on the term 'similar' because there are a lot of incorrect definitions that refer to endo as the endometrium, despite histological and genetic variations. If we want more awareness for this condition, we gotta make sure everyone is across the right description—so, say it with me, endometriosis is not the endometrium! The difference between the cells that form in the uterine lining and these cells that are found *outside* the uterus is that the innies have an exit point each month—our period. But the outies have nowhere to go! They just stay there, thickening with each month that passes and can lead to the formation of adhesions and endometriomas, aka 'chocolate cysts'. Not sure what they are?

Adhesions are bands of scar tissue that can bind organs together and create a different kind of pain that some consider to be a sharp or tugging sensation.

Endometriomas are fluid-filled sacs/pockets in an ovary or on its surface and are often called 'chocolate cysts' which sounds kinda yum but it's not really because the fluid is old (dark) blood.

While the most common place for endometriosis to occur is within the pelvic cavity and on reproductive organs, it is still regarded as a whole-body disease because it can be found in other places too. Endometriosis can be classified as:

→ **Endopelvic**—lesser/minor pelvis, ovaries, fallopian tubes, recto-uterine pouch and ligaments posterior of the uterus

→ **Extrapelvic**—pretty much all disease found outside the reproductive organs. We're talking abdominal wall, scars of the perineum (between the anus and vulva), the urinary and gastrointestinal tract, the thorax, brain and even the lining of the nasal cavity (nasal mucosa if you want to get fancy)

→ **Thoracic**—chest cavity, diaphragm, lungs

→ **Sciatic**—sciatic nerve, which branches from your lower back through your hips and butt and down each leg.

So, what does endometriosis look like? A common assumption is that the disease is purely of a dark appearance, but the lesions can come in all sorts of colours such as white, red, yellow, brown and even clear. They can be thick and they can also be as fine as strand of hair but unfortunately, not all gynaecologists and specialists have the skills to correctly identify all forms of endometriosis.

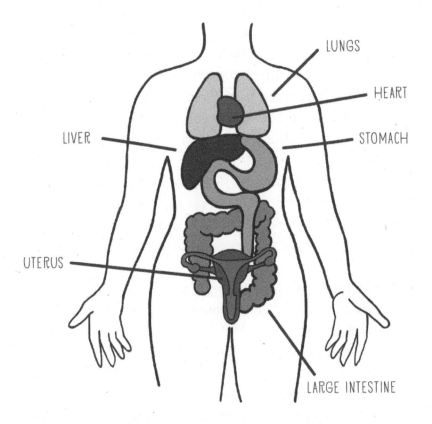

Endo is a whole-body disease

Whether it's superficial or deep infiltrating, endo is BRUTAL. In 2019, the National Health Service (UK) listed endometriosis as one of the top twenty most painful health conditions— endo pain can be so disabling it can inhibit daily tasks. Endo was named alongside the likes of fibromyalgia, heart attacks and broken bones. It can be so damaging that some people may require an ileostomy bag (an external pouching system that collects intestinal waste), a walking aid or a wheelchair. If that doesn't give you an idea as to how hectic this condition can be, here's some ways in which my endogram followers have described their pain.

- *'Like two knives stabbing into my uterus.'*
- *'A cheese grater in my uterus.'*
- *'Like my ovaries and fallopian tubes are being twisted and pricked with needles.'*
- *'Red hot coal burning inside my guts.'*
- *'A chainsaw across your uterus and lower back.'*
- *'Sitting on a knife with pain shooting up through my bowel and to my belly button.'*
- *'Burning, like someone is holding a lighter to my insides.'*
- *'Like a bowling ball being dropped on to my pelvis.'*
- *'It's as if I'm birthing barbed wire.'*
- *'Feels like my organs are being twisted and squeezed.'*

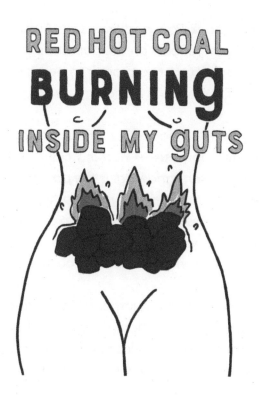

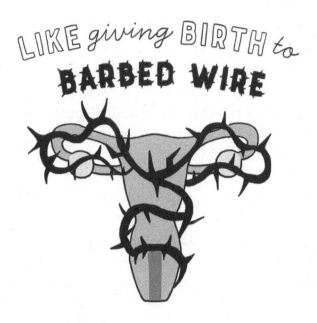

LIKE giving BIRTH to BARBED WIRE

In her 2019 book *Pain and Prejudice*, Australian journalist Gabrielle Jackson reflects on the pain she's endured over the years, ranging from a broken back to being hit by a train in India. Yep, HIT BY A TRAIN. She says:

> But this pain—this pain after the laparoscopy and the pain of endometriosis—is nothing like that. This ache, this always present gnawing, is the pain that makes me feel bad. No painkiller puts me in a happy mood with this pain. No bliss overcomes me. No drug can stop the nausea once it arrives. Only stillness helps. But stillness is so hard. I've felt ten, and I can tell you, this pain is worse.

But wait, there's more! Another super fun fact about endo is that there is no prevention, no cure and no determined cause. There are a few theories floating around but none can fully explain why endometriosis occurs and, due to the lack of evidence, I'm not going to include them in this book—I don't think it helps. According to the Center for Endometriosis Care, it is likely that a number of factors including genetic/epigenetic predispositions play significant roles in determining which, when and whether an individual will develop this condition. The main thing to know is that it is NOT your fault. You don't have endometriosis because you did or didn't do something.

Endometriosis affects one in ten people assigned female at birth and in a national study of 13,508 Australian cisgender women, one in nine were diagnosed with endometriosis by age 44. There are more than approximately 800,000 endo warriors in Australia, around 1.5 million in the UK, and worldwide, the estimation is at least 176 million. Experts call endometriosis the 'silent epidemic'. However, it's not just a women's health issue. Endo can affect teens as well as transgender and non-binary people and, in rare cases, cisgender men.

You'll notice that I refer to endo sufferers as people with endometriosis. Unfortunately, due to the lack of awareness and research on this condition, it is difficult to speak author-itatively on behalf of transgender and non-binary sufferers who have been excluded from research studies. Any data in this book is based on cisgender women (unless stated otherwise) but I hope that, moving forward, research will be more inclusive and representative. We have a *long* way to go in terms of how we can help gender-diverse people navigate their health and I will be reflecting on that later in the book.

What are the symptoms?

Well . . . there are a cheeky few.

A common misconception is that endometriosis is just bad periods, but it is *so much more than that*. In fact, one of the biggest complexities of this condition is the varying range of symptoms and how individualised they are. Everyone experiences endo differently and my pain may not match yours or vice versa. There are even people out there who don't experience any symptoms of endo! Alongside heavy/irregular bleeding and pain connected to ovulation, the abdomen, back and pelvis, some common symptoms include:

Pain when emptying the bladder

This is one of my biggest symptoms—it turns out that endo implants on the bladder can cause inflammation and muscle tension, resulting in painful pees. And do you ever feel like you have twenty litres of urine ready to go, but it ends up only being a few drops? That's the story of my life, and it's due to hypersensitivity of the nerves.

Pain during or after sex

When there's thrusting or penetration during intercourse, the endometrial implants in the pelvic cavity can stretch, pull or push. And it bloody hurts, fam! It is not pleasant. It also doesn't help that our bodies respond to this pain by clenching up which in turn promotes more pain. The number of nerves multiply, it's all too sensitive and what should feel good, doesn't. We'll touch on this in more detail later in the book.

Fatigue

As noted by the Endometriosis Foundation of America, the main cause of endometriosis-related fatigue is the body's effort to eliminate the diseased tissue. While the immune system attempts to combat endo, cytokines (aka inflammatory toxins) are secreted by the tissue. What we feel to be fatigue is the result of these internal chemicals. A particularly shitty thing about endo fatigue is that it tends to go unnoticed as a symptom. There's definitely stigma and an assumption that it's not legitimate because it's technically not pain—but fatigue is not just being tired, either. We are talking about a constant lack of energy due to the internal battles our bodies are fighting and something that not even a good night's rest can solve.

Pain during bowel movements

Speaking of shitty! Did you know that endometriosis has a direct relationship with our gastrointestinal tract? Also referred to as our gut, the GI functions as the centre of our body's digestive system. It's where our large intestine, colon, small intestine, small bowel and rectum sit together. Endo implants on or near the GI tract can not only trigger muscle tension and painful bowel movements but also diarrhoea, constipation, nausea and . . .

Abdominal bloating

Aka endo belly. Endo causes scar tissue that can bind up the abdominal organs and slow down the intestines. On top of this, endometriosis lesions can flare up at different times throughout the menstrual cycle, causing an immune response which creates swelling. For some people, this swelling can be so intense that they look pregnant which is a pretty cruel irony . . .

Infertility

We will explore this later in the book but, in short, studies show that there are two ways in which endo may affect fertility. One being its inflammatory power preventing a suitable environment for egg fertilisation. The other suggests a more structural issue in that our anatomy can be distorted through scar tissue and adhesions, potentially causing the blockage of fallopian tubes.

What's with the stages of endometriosis?

Endo has been classified into four stages by the American Society of Reproductive Medicine to measure the physical presence of the disease. It is super important to highlight, however, that these stages of endometriosis have been determined based on the impact on fertility and spread of lesions; they do not reflect the level of pain or presence of symptoms. For example, I was diagnosed with stage four which means I had A LOT of endo spread across various spots, but I've never passed out from my pain, nor has it prevented me from holding down a full-time job. However, I know people who often black out from their flare-ups and cannot commit to full-time work due to their debilitating pain, and they're a stage two or three. The American Society for Reproductive Medicine also use a weighted point system but as someone who dropped maths in Year 10, I am *completely* thrown off whenever I see numbers. I find this stage-by-stage breakdown easier to follow.

- **Stage one**—minimal with few superficial implants
- **Stage two**—mild with more frequent and deeper implants
- **Stage three**—moderate with many deep implants, as well as small cysts on one or both ovaries and the presence of filmy adhesions
- **Stage four**—severe with many deep implants, as well as large cysts on one or both ovaries and many dense adhesions.

The stages are good to refer to when you receive your diagnosis but, again, they absolutely do not factor in or reflect the pain and/or symptoms that you endure. I personally disagree with measuring your endo experience according to this framework as it can invalidate those in the earlier stages. We need a staging system that factors in the severity of symptoms and the impact endo can have on your life.

So, what's being done about endometriosis?

Endometriosis is as common as asthma and diabetes yet it falls so far behind in terms of awareness, research and funding. In 2016, the Australian National Health and Medical Research Council (NHMRC) allocated $14.7 million to asthma research, $64.1 million to diabetes research and $837,433 to endometriosis research. Why such a difference? Well, here's what I'm seeing. I'm seeing two conditions that are known to affect 'everyone', and another that is regarded as just a cisgender women's health issue. This isn't an isolated issue.

From heart disease to chronic pain, research has always been based on the anatomy of a cisgender man. Since literally *forever,* women's pain has been downplayed in the world of medicine and healthcare. Just google 'hysteria' and you'll see what I mean. Even in terms of research, it was as recently as 2013 that a case study was published where the research question was to consider physical attractiveness in women with and without endometriosis. Physical attractiveness. You couldn't possibly find something more distasteful, tone-deaf and irrelevant. At the 2019 RANZCOG (Royal Australian and New Zealand College of Obstetricians and Gynaecologists) Annual Scientific Meeting, Professor Peter Rogers (University of Melbourne, Royal Women's Hospital) advocated for a change in priorities to aid endometriosis research. 'We are way behind in terms of clinical trials and the capacity and resources to do them,' he claimed.

Despite that, there has been promising progress for recognition of endometriosis. In 2016, a groundbreaking documentary called *Endo What?* was released to high acclaim from all over the world. The following year, Irish author Sally Rooney published her debut novel *Conversations With Friends*, with her fictional female protagonist suffering from endo. The National Action Plan for Endometriosis, rolled out by the Australian Government Department of Health in 2018, was designed to improve public awareness of endometriosis, patients' understanding of the condition, treatment options and research programs into endometriosis and chronic pelvic pain. We've seen public figures like Lena Dunham, Halsey and Emma Watkins (Emma Wiggle) step up to share their own endo journeys along with millions of people using social media as a tool for conversation and advocacy. Patients have taken it upon themselves to lead for change and, to be frank, it is bloody inspiring.

Think of endometriosis as a big and often frustrating puzzle. There's never a clear starting point and piecing it together takes a lot of time and patience. Sometimes you will definitely want to just flip the whole thing and walk away. The puzzle isn't complete and sometimes I wonder if it ever will be—yet we persist, uncovering its connections and patterns along the way.

Endo myths—BUSTED!

Look, there's a lot of BS floating around regarding endometriosis. Lots of theories, lots of misinterpretation and a whole lotta myths. So, let's set the record straight on a few things.

Hysterectomy does NOT cure endo

Endometriosis is tissue *similar* to the lining of the uterus, that grows *outside* of the uterus. Therefore, removing the uterus will *not* remove the endo. It may relieve some symptoms, but it won't cure endo. Why? Because there is no cure for endo!

Pregnancy does NOT cure endo

Some people with endometriosis may experience temporary suppression of their symptoms while pregnant but, again, there is no cure for endo! Also, it's pretty cooked to suggest this to someone with endo given that infertility is a particularly devastating symptom for a number of people, so can we stop doing that?

Teenagers CAN get endo

Prior to the introduction of laparoscopy in the 1970s, endometriosis could only be diagnosed during a laparotomy, which is a major surgical procedure resulting in some decent-sized scars. We're talking a ten to fifteen centimetre incision into the abdomen, so pretty gnarly stuff. Because of the risks and costs associated with a laparotomy, this procedure was only really performed as a last resort for those with super severe symptoms, who were past child-bearing age. So, obviously, not teens. Nobody is too young to have this condition and it's often throughout adolescence that our symptoms develop—even though many of us won't receive a diagnosis until we're in our twenties or thirties. Endometriosis has even been found in unborn foetuses!

Menopause does NOT stop endo

As you probably know, menopause is when you stop menstruating. The body's production of estrogen and progesterone slows down and your hormone levels fall to a point where your ovaries stop releasing eggs. However, there is no guarantee that menopause will stop your endo because the lesions create *their own* localised estrogen.

Birth control does NOT stop endo

Birth control can treat the symptoms of endo, but there's no evidence to suggest it can treat or stop the growth of the actual disease itself. I know birth control has relieved pain for some people, which is awesome and each to their own, but it's important to remember that it is there serving as a bandaid.

Endometriosis is NOT a menstrual disease

One of the proposed theories surrounding endometriosis is this thing called retrograde menstruation, which is when blood flows backwards into the pelvis instead of out of the vagina during menstruation. However, the problem with this theory is that regardless of whether you menstruate or not, endo's gonna endo. It does not grow in accordance to menstrual cycles and, as mentioned previously, endo has been found in people who do not have uteruses; therefore, it cannot be regarded as a menstrual disease or a disease of the uterus. Why? Because . . .

Endometriosis is NOT the endometrium

Therefore, it doesn't always correspond to the usual hormonal changes that induce menstruation. Honestly, I feel bad for all the hate and resentment directed towards the uterus. Endo is in a different lane and the uterus is not to blame!

" It is imperative to look beyond gendered health and include all people in endometriosis, many of whom are already struggling to access diagnosis, quality treatment and supportive care in a traditionally female-identified space. **"**

CENTER FOR ENDOMETRIOSIS CARE

2

Diagnosis

Endometriosis is a tricky name to pronounce but it's even harder to diagnose. How hard? According to new research from Endometriosis Australia, it takes an average of six and a half years. I always thought it took me six years but if we actually base it on the first time that I approached a doctor with period concerns, which was in 2006, it would be double that. Twelve years! It can be a little sad to look at my life in that time frame. Don't get me wrong, my life has been very good. I've travelled, fallen in love and, all in all, I am really proud of what I have achieved. Yet, I can't help but think how many times over these past twelve years I have felt extremely limited by this condition. How many times I've curled up in agony, how many painkillers I've taken or how many hours I have spent staring aimlessly into the microwave as my heat pack warms up on a Saturday night while everyone else is out. I've pushed these thoughts to the back of my mind but when they do seep through, it's a little melancholic, imagining how much better my quality of life could have been if my diagnosis was made earlier.

So, why the heck does it take so long to diagnose endo?! It's a big, valid and frustrating question that has several answers beyond the obvious lack of recognition, education and awareness for the disease.

Society has normalised pain, but not periods

Does that heading make you want to scream into a pillow? Because same. As we have learned, endometriosis isn't just a bad period but that is usually the first red flag. A big problem here is that there is no frame of reference for menstruators to compare our pain to—we've always been told it's just how they are and that we should suck it up. A study in Austria and Germany found that normalisation of period pain means that menstruators often wait two to three years from the onset of symptoms before consulting a medical professional.

We want to talk about our pain but because of the social stigmas attached, we choose pain over shame.

Attitudes of health professionals

This is a big one. I'm definitely not saying all health professionals are bad but, frankly, too many have failed us. I mean, we are talking about a system that historically has been rooted in sexist notions of women's hysteria. To take just one famous example, English doctor Isaac Baker Brown surgically removed the clitorises of thousands of women as a cure for insanity, epilepsy and hysteria.

I can't believe I'm about to refer to Reddit in my debut book but 2020 has proved that anything and everything could happen, so here we are. As I write this, a screenshot from Reddit is currently going viral:

Again, it's from Reddit so I can't 1000 per cent verify it and anxiety *is* a real condition, but the devastating reality is that anyone with endometriosis reading this would not be surprised. At all. I believe it! I believe it based on the twelve years it took me to get an answer for my pain. I believe it based on *your* pain. I believe it based on, basically, all of the above!

Symptoms are often mistaken for other conditions

When you experience pain during sex, you're more likely to be tested for a UTI than for endo. Period pain is usually passed off as dysmenorrhea without further investigation into endo or adenomyosis. Bloating? It's just Irritable Bowel Syndrome. All legitimate things but the problem with many medical professionals is that they don't look *beyond* these conditions. Nor do many connect the dots and consider the whole-body effects of endometriosis.

There is no simple or straightforward way to test for endometriosis

Currently, the only definitive way to obtain a pathological diagnosis for endo is by laparoscopic excision surgery. Surgery being the only true form of detection is a barrier for many reasons. Not everyone can afford time off for surgery, nor can everyone afford the surgery itself. There could also be extended wait times, depending on whether you go through the private or public health system and where you live (i.e. rural or metro). It's a bit of a hot mess, but we will explore other ways in which endo can be detected shortly.

Seeking a diagnosis for endometriosis is particularly chaotic because where do you even start? There is no step-by-step handbook out there to guide us along this confusing and daunting path, so it's hard not to feel completely paralysed like a deer in headlights. But that's why I'm here! Let this book steer you across that dangerous road as we follow a more promising route together.

Before we take off, we need to pack. And while snacks are always a good idea, I'm talking about packing some sweet, sweet knowledge! Our first stop is the GP's office to refer us on to a specialist, but I wouldn't leave it to them to decide you who see. Unless your GP is a total legend and has already flexed some expertise regarding endo, I highly recommend doing your own research on which specialist you would like to take on your case.

When I say specialist, I'm not referring to an obstetrician-gynaecologist. Yes, an OB-GYN specialises in two things that concern endometriosis, being pregnancy and reproductive health, however they may not necessarily have the sufficient training to surgically detect and remove endo. You'll hear more about this procedure in the next chapter but to put it simply, endo is *not* simple! You ideally want to see a specialist whose work revolves around this disease, not someone who's delivering babies at all sorts of hours and then scrubbing in to check out some endo. That may come across as dismissive but it's the truth: this condition requires full-time investment and not all OB-GYNs have completed the advanced training and fellowships that are required for treating endo.

Endometriosis specialists

It's not easy to find an endo specialist and it requires a lot of research, but thanks mainly to the advocacy of the patient community, this information is more accessible than ever before. A good place to start would be your local online support group where you can read through posts from others who have outlined their experiences and offered recommendations. Another would be Nancy's Nook Endometriosis Education, which is a private Facebook group and also a website (you'll find the details in the Recommended Resources section). After doing this, I would then have a good suss out on the internet to see if the recommended specialist you've found has a website and what information is available regarding their qualifications and training.

At the very least, they should have a fellowship in minimally invasive gynaecology surgery and accreditation with the relevant body, such as AGES (Australian Gynaecological Endoscopy and Surgical Society) or RANZCOG (Royal Australian and New Zealand College of Obstetricians and Gynaecologists).

In 2019, committees from both bodies signed off on guidelines for performing gynaecological endoscopic procedures. While the information doesn't serve as an official assessment, it's such a handy document that we can access (for free!) online to help gain a better sense of our consulting professional's level of experience.

For example, a true specialist should have accreditation and credentialing in Level 6 Scope of Clinical Practice with RANZCOG. Level 6 indicates they have been trained in excising stage one to four endometriosis. Whereas Level 1 only indicates training in ablation surgery.

One tool that has been designed to help streamline the process of finding the right specialist is iCareBetter. It basically serves as an endometriosis specialist directory where surgeons who wish to be listed need to pass a vigorous reviewing process that evaluates their surgical and excision skills. It's currently available in the United States but there are plans to extend it throughout multiple countries and continents so there's real potential for it to be a worldwide game changer for the patient community.

Once you've done your checking around and have decided on a specialist you would like to see, it's time to take that request to the GP's office. And I truly pray you do not have the same experience that I did with old mate who told me flat out that I didn't have endo.

This step can be pretty daunting because you do feel like you have to justify yourself—it's almost as if you're presenting a pitch. Like, we have to convince them to believe us? Shouldn't they just . . . believe us?

Come with receipts

Have you ever walked into a medical consult feeling super confident but when it's your turn to speak, nothing comes out? Your mind blanks? This has happened to me plenty of times, but one thing I have found super helpful is bringing in my receipts! I don't mean your supermarket dockets, I mean receipts in the form of previous scans, a pain diary, study papers and any research you think applies to your case. Go in with guns blazing!

Diarise your symptoms

A pain diary is going to make it so easy for you to answer some of the GP's questions. You can do this the old-fashioned way with a pen and notepad, or perhaps there's an app out there that you already use to track period-related symptoms, so why not incorporate your endo symptoms? In June 2020, Australian organisation QENDO launched a free app for those suffering with endometriosis, adenomyosis, polycystic ovary syndrome or chronic pelvic pain. I highly recommend downloading this one as it allows you to rate your pain and describe your period—you can track everything!

Take notes

I don't know about you, but too many times I have left a medical consult only to forget what was said. It can be really hard to retain all the important information that they are providing, so ask if you can take notes. Sometimes we're too scared to do this and worried that it might offend the doctor or strike a blow to their ego. It's really just how you word it with them—try something like: 'If you don't mind, I'd really love to take some notes as this is really important to me and I value what you have to say. I want to make sure I can check the details when I get home.'

Back yourself

Medical consults are intimidating at the best of times but they're even more scary when it's concerning an invisible illness. It doesn't matter how many medical professionals you deal with and it doesn't matter how much experience they have, YOU are the expert of your own body. No-one else. You live in this body, day in, day out. You know it better than anyone else. Plus, you have rights! When you walk into that consultation room, you are in control and the GP is there to help YOU. You are entitled to know all the risks and benefits of all treatment options put forward. You also have every right to refuse any treatment method or procedure that you are uncomfortable with.

Listen to your gut

If the doctor doesn't feel like the right fit, chances are they're not. Go find someone else. There is a systemic distrust of doctors within the endometriosis community—and for good reason—but they're not all the same. Finding an expert doctor can be difficult at times, but it doesn't mean you should stick around with a bad one.

There are also a number of tools available to help GPs and patients, such as:

→ **Diagnosis and Management of Endometriosis in New Zealand**—a publication developed by a taskforce of representatives from the New Zealand Ministry of Health, RANZCOG, the Royal New Zealand College of General Practitioners (RNZCGP), the Faculty of Pain Medicine of the Australian and New Zealand College of Anaesthetists (FPMANZCA), Endometriosis New Zealand and those who live with endometriosis. It's not a formal clinical guideline, but it provides a consensus view of best-practice principles that aim to improve the diagnosis and management of endometriosis in New Zealand in primary and secondary healthcare.

→ **Raising Awareness Tool for Endometriosis (RATE)**— an accessible electronic resource designed to help health professionals and patients identify and assess endometriosis and endometriosis-associated symptoms. RATE was developed by gynaecologists, general practitioners, pain medicine specialists, fertility specialists, emergency physicians and nurses working with RANZCOG.

→ **The Pain Perception Project, by Ohnut.co and Duvet Days**—a patient-founded initiative producing various tools for better understanding pain, starting with an online Pelvic Pain Assessment that helps patients effectively communicate their symptoms with doctors.

Seeing your specialist

You'll need to repeat a few of the things you said when speaking with your GP. Bring your medical history, pain diary and take notes. You'll want to ask a few more questions because it's important to establish whether or not you feel good moving forward with this specialist.

Here are a few to help you get started (but honestly, there could be 100,000 more!):

- What is your training and fellowship background?
- Can you tell me more about the appearance of endo?
- How many endometriosis cases do you deal with annually?
- What is your success rate in terms of patients returning for additional surgeries?
- What is your preferred method of removing endometriosis and why? (See Chapter 3!)
- Where do you stand on hormonal treatment for endometriosis? (See Chapter 3!)
- What is your post-op approach in terms of ongoing management of the condition?
- Do you work alongside others who specialise in other areas of the body that endo may be found (that is, a colorectal surgeon, a urologist, a cardiothoracic surgeon, etc)?
- Do you operate in both public and private hospital settings?
- Do you have a waitlist?
- What would you recommend for pain management while I wait for a surgical diagnosis?

If you are not satisfied with how your questions are answered, seek a second opinion. It may seem daunting, but it can have a huge pay-off. Just ask Brooklynn Chess, my endo mate from Seattle who runs the Instagram account @the_endo_chronic_ills. It took ten years for Brooklynn to receive her endo diagnosis and, even then, she was misinformed by her first gynaecologist, who insisted on combining a gonadotropin-releasing hormone receptor (GnRH) such as Lupron or Orilissa with an antidepressant as treatment. Brooklynn trusted her gynaecologist and agreed to a diagnostic laparoscopy. Despite detecting stage three endometriosis, Brooklynn's gynaecologist decided against removing the disease and continued to endorse these drugs, claiming they would stop Brooklynn's endometriosis from progressing any further. Brooklynn told me:

> There were many factors that contributed to my decision to seek a second opinion. I had pretty much always put my faith in my medical team and listened to their recommendations, but when my first doctor repeatedly downplayed my symptoms and made me feel as though they were all in my head—then diagnosed me with endometriosis that was too difficult for her to treat— I knew there had to be better options for me, and thus far nobody had helped me, so I decided to take more control of my diagnosis and medical care.

Brooklynn turned to Nancy's Nook on Facebook where she learned about excision surgery and immediately started searching for a specialist. After considering four options, Brooklynn decided on The Center for Endometriosis Care in Atlanta, Georgia, and it changed everything.

> When I first spoke to my endometriosis specialist, I instantly felt validated and understood. He never down-played my symptoms or made me feel like it was in my head. Prior to surgery I received a forty-page pre-op

packet and was directed to the Center for Endometriosis Care's website which contains a plethora of useful and educational information that I still refer back to, to this day. I think I had tears in my eyes the whole time during my pre-op appointment because it was the first time in my life that I was in a healthcare setting where I was actually understood.

Brooklynn underwent excision surgery alongside other procedures (video-assisted thoracoscopic surgery (VATS), appendectomy, cystoscopy, hysteroscopy and chromotubation) and received a detailed diagnosis of widespread endometriosis that her first gynaecologist was unable to do. She was provided with post-operation photos and her post-op report was fifteen pages long. Seeking a second opinion was the best decision she ever made.

Once you've found a specialist you're happy with, the next step they will likely take is to talk through some methods that can help confirm suspicions of endo.

Manual pelvic exam

Your specialist may want to perform a manual pelvic exam which involves them feeling around areas within your pelvis for cysts or signs of scar tissue. This allows them to check for pain, tenderness and any ovarian abnormalities. Your specialist should always ask for consent first and you should not feel pressured to agree to this examination if you do not feel comfortable.

Ultrasound

As you probably know, an ultrasound is an imaging method in which soundwaves are used to produce pictures of the inside of the body. An ultrasound technician, called a sonographer, will apply a special lubricating jelly to your skin. This prevents friction so they can rub the ultrasound transducer on your skin. The transducer sends high-frequency soundwaves through your body, which echo as they hit an organ or bone. Those echoes are then recorded by a computer to form a picture that can be interpreted by the doctor.

A standard transvaginal ultrasound is an internal ultrasound which involves observing the pelvic area by scanning it with an ultrasound probe placed just inside the vagina. Your specialist might ask for a DIE (deep infiltrating endometriosis) scan which is a more thorough ultrasound. Superficial lesions of endometriosis can never be diagnosed on ultrasound as they have no real mass, only colour.

MRI

Magnetic resonance imaging is a scan that uses strong magnetic fields, radio waves and a computer to take pictures of the soft tissue inside of your body, but not all endo can be detected through an MRI scan.

Depending on your situation, you may be asked to bowel prep for an ultrasound and MRI. Bowel preparation is a bowel cleanse with a laxative drink, tablets and/or enema. I have done only one bowel prep before a DIE scan using a fleet enema. It's a clear liquid in a bottle, you insert the nozzle into your butt and squirt the full contents of the bottle into the rectum. It is awkward and uncomfortable but ya gotta do what ya gotta do.

Sometimes a diagnosis can be suggested based on these tests but there is no definitive way to know without having a laparoscopy.

Your specialist may also want to prescribe some pain medication and suggest some other pain management techniques such as:

Heat relief

You know the term 'crazy cat lady'? That's me but with heat packs. I have a whole bathroom drawer dedicated to my warm little friends. These glorious sacks are instant comfort. Well, after a few minutes in the microwave they are. Alternatively, you can try stick-on heat pads or an electric heating blanket.

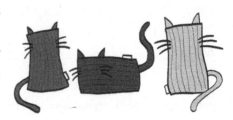

TENS machine

Another drug-free form of relief that people with endometriosis turn to is a Transcutaneous Electrical Nerve Stimulator (TENS) machine. These are small, unobtrusive machines with electrodes that attach to the skin and send electrical pulses into the body. The pulses do not hurt, they're more of a mild

tickle and they're supposed
to work by either blocking
the pain messages as they
travel through the nerves
or by helping the body
produce endorphins which
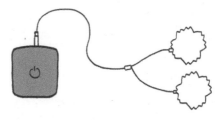
are natural pain-fighters. TENS machines vary in price and
size and some can be clipped to a belt. Personally, I'm yet to
have any luck with them relieving my pain, but it's different
for everybody.

Birth control

There are various forms of birth control such as the Pill, IUDs
and contraceptive implants that can help suppress your
symptoms but there is no evidence to suggest that birth
control will stop your endo from growing back. It's entirely up
to you as to whether you want to try them, just remember
to be fully informed about the potential risks and know
that, in terms of endometriosis, birth control merely serves
as a bandaid.

Be cautious of GnRH drugs too, like what Brooklynn was
offered by her gynaecologist in the form of Lupron and
Orilissa. They don't do anything to prevent endo from growing
back and can present some serious side effects, so make
sure you do your research before deciding on any treatment.
Remember, hormonal suppression is symptom management
and that is not the same thing as actually treating endometriosis and its progression as a disease.

"They now have chewable Viagra. But they can't throw us a bone with endometriosis?"

AMY SCHUMER

3

Surgery and recovery

As we have covered already, the way in which endometriosis is surgically detected and removed is through a laparoscopic procedure. A laparoscopy, also known as keyhole surgery, is where a surgical telescope and video camera is passed through a small cut, a 'keyhole' in the abdomen, usually in the belly button. The patient is placed under general anaesthetic and their abdomen is inflated with carbon dioxide gas so the pelvic organs are clearly visible and operable. Instruments can be passed through one or more other small cuts in the wall of the abdomen, which are referred to as incision points and are usually about one centimetre in length. Alongside the removal of endometriosis, a laparoscopy can be used to treat scar tissue as well as assessing fertility and functionality of fallopian tubes and ovaries. Your specialist should communicate which procedures they plan on undertaking, the purpose of each and hopefully they help you pronounce them too, because we are dealing with words that are Big and Technical. To give you an idea, this is what I had done during my second laparoscopy, in addition to excision of endometriosis:

- **Tubal patency**—tests whether fallopian tubes are open or not
- **Neurolysis**—surgical application of physical or chemical agents to a nerve to cause a temporary degeneration of targeted nerve fibres, relieving neurological symptoms resulting from nerve infiltration by endometriosis
- **Oophoropexy**—surgical technique that utilises a dissolving suture to temporarily suspend the ovaries away from the pelvic sidewall, to which they might otherwise adhere to in the post-op period
- **Adhesiolysis**—surgical procedure to divide adhesions that are fusing organs together
- **Hysteroscopy**—surgical procedure in which a small camera is inserted through the cervix to examine the uterus
- **D and C (Dilatation and Curettage)**—where a sample of the lining is removed and sent for analysis
- **IUD removal**—pretty straightforward, removing IUD from uterus.

If your gynaecologist/specialist has recommended surgery, they also need to tell you about the two ways in which endometriosis and scar tissue is removed—ablation and excision. Unfortunately, it's not often that patients will be told any of this and it wasn't until after my first laparoscopy that I became aware of the two methods! If they don't raise it, you are within your rights to ask because you really do need to know which one they are using and the reason behind that choice. Why is it so important, you may wonder? Well, it turns out that the technique has a huge influence on a lot of things like recurrence of endo, recovery and how you deal with pain moving forward.

Ablation

Ablation uses heat energy to burn/vaporise the endometrial cells. Ablation is generally more accessible and less expensive but that's because it requires less training than excision, therefore more gynaecologists can do it. That may sound beneficial but it's actually quite concerning because not all gynaecologists specialise in endometriosis, especially its removal. Think of ablation as like burning the leaves off weeds. It eliminates that top layer, but it leaves behind everything else like the root and other scar tissue—and therefore the recurrence rate of endometriosis growing back is high. Because of this, deep infiltrating endometriosis cannot be sufficiently removed by ablation and, because of the nature of the procedure, there is also no way to obtain a specimen for true pathological diagnosis. The number of stories I have heard from people in online support groups who have had multiple ablations without knowing the real information is heartbreaking. In the incredible book *Beating Endo*, Dr Iris Kerin Orbuch recalls one patient who had gone through nineteen (NINETEEN!) ablation procedures, each bringing mild relief for a brief period of time. Little did this patient realise that these surgeries weren't to treat returning endometriosis, but in fact the endo had simply never left in the first place. Its core and root remained while the surface continued to be skimmed over and over again.

A quick note on endometrial ablation: this is something that may or may not pop up throughout your endo journey. Endometrial ablation is a different procedure to the ablation of endometriosis as it is primarily used to treat heavy period bleeding by burning the uterine lining. However, it does little for endo pain because endometriosis is not the endometrium. Endometrial ablation should also not be used on people who are pregnant or those who plan to conceive. Consult your specialist for more information.

Excision

Although not a cure, excision is deemed the gold standard when it comes to treating endometriosis as it surgically removes the entire lesion from its root. This can be done with surgical tools, a laser used as a knife and through robotic assistance. You know how I likened ablation to burning the leaves off weeds? Excision is like a trowel that physically cuts the whole of it out. This way, surrounding organs are less likely to be damaged or removed and the chance of recurrence is significantly lower than with ablation. However, due to the more invasive nature of excision as opposed to ablation, specialists are required to undertake more study and training to be able to perform it. For this reason, finding an excision specialist can be harder than hitting up a regular OB-GYN. Not only that, expect a longer recovery time.

Excision allows for pathological diagnosis of the disease and while it may be harder and more expensive to seek, the sheer precision is *so* worth it. An easy way to remember excision as the superior method is with a good old alliteration. Excision = excellent.

Or, check out this analogy by Dr Abhishek Mangeshikar, the founder and director of The Indian Centre for Endometriosis (ICE), who likens the treatment of endometriosis to a splinter. A patient walks into the offices of various doctors, seeking advice on this painful condition.

- **Doctor 1:** Take these pills, they should sort out the pain (medical therapy)
- **Doctor 2:** There's no splinter, it's all in your head (medical gaslighting)
- **Doctor 3:** I'm just going to burn off the top of the splinter and that will take care of the problem (ablation)
- **Doctor 4:** I think we need to remove the entire finger (hysterectomy)
- **Doctor 5:** We need to remove the splinter in its entirety, including the root embedded in the flesh (excision)

I don't know about you, but I think I'll be hitting up Doctor 5.

Leading up to your procedure

There are a few things you can be doing in the lead-up to your procedure that will help improve your recovery. You should seek specific advice from your surgeon as they may have some additional instructions such as bowel prep, but here are some general tips to get you started:

- stop smoking
- abstain from alcohol
- try to do at least two weeks of daily gentle exercise (even if it's a thirty-minute walk every day)
- practise pelvic stretches and deep breathing exercises
- try to maintain a healthy diet of fresh vegetables and ·fruits, etc
- drink lots of water and . . .

Stay calm! The lead-up to surgery can be daunting for many reasons. Perhaps you fear the idea of being put to sleep or maybe you are worried that they won't find anything. These feelings are totally valid and we all go through it. I have been placed under general anaesthetic ten times now for various procedures and I still get scared! I think what really helps is just accepting that you can't control everything and whatever happens, you will be able to handle it like the boss you are. Any concerns you have, your surgeon and anaesthetist are there to help. You might like to ask:

- What is the expected duration of my procedure?
- How much time off work/study do you anticipate I will need to take?
- What will you do if endo is found somewhere you were not expecting it? Will there be other specialists available to assist or would we look at addressing this in a separate surgery?

- Will there be anyone in training who may operate or is it just you?
- How soon after my procedure will I see you?

Be sure to also share any concerns regarding painkillers and possible nausea, in case they need adjust your planned prescriptions. For additional support, I recommend seeking an online endo group in your area.

What to pack for hospital

Even if you are booked in as a day procedure, it's still a good idea to pack a bag in case they decide to keep you overnight. This happened for my first surgery, I was supposed to be in and out but due to the severity of my endo, they wanted to keep me in for monitoring. I didn't have a problem with that but, boy, it was *not* easy trying to tell my partner where he could find my belongings around my share house. Because we were doing long distance, he obviously had no idea where anything was in my bedroom and, honestly, giving instructions is the last thing you want to do when you are riding that trippy anaesthetic wave. Learn from my lack of preparation! Some important things to pack include:

- ID, bank cards, health insurance information
- phone charger
- pads (you will be too sore for tampons and sometimes the hospital only give you cardboard-like pads, so pack some from your favourite brand)
- comfortable, loose-fitting underwear and PJs

- comfortable, loose-fitting clothes to wear home (trackies and a button-up shirt are super easy to put on)
- slip-on shoes (that is, thongs or sandals) for showering and for wearing home. Last thing you'll wanna deal with is shoelaces!
- hairbrush and hair elastics
- toothbrush, toothpaste, floss, deodorant
- heat pack and/or stick-on head pads (in case they cannot provide heated towels for your stomach)
- earplugs and eye mask (in case you're in a shared room)
- headphones
- download music and TV shows onto your phone (in case your room does not have a TV).

What to have at home

- Someone to help you! You shouldn't be doing any housework—no cooking or washing
- Comfy pillows including a tri pillow for extra back support and a small one to pop on your stomach when sneezing/coughing
- Heat packs, for your stomach AND your shoulders!
- Peppermint tea and De-Gas/Gasx capsules to help relieve any shoulder tip gas pain
- Regular painkillers and any post-op prescribed medication—talk to your specialist about this
- Pre-prepared meals (you'll need to avoid exerting yourself following surgery), soft foods like soup, smoothies, salads and steamed veggies, etc
- Walking stick and shower chair if you need

- Plenty of water because hydration is always essential, especially for speeding up the healing process
- Comfortable sheets: you'll need to rest!

Recovery

So you're fresh outta surgery, rocking some new scars and a tender, bloated belly. You're feeling pretty floaty from the drugs and you've probably got a million questions swirling around in that hazy brain of yours. Your surgeon may visit you in recovery or the next day if you are required to stay overnight. They may even advise that you will receive the information in your post-op consultation which is usually in the weeks following your procedure and, if that happens, I would hold my ground and persist for some sort of detail because screw having to wait a few weeks! Here are a few questions you may like to consider asking in addition to any others you have planned:

- How long did my procedure take?
- Did you find any endometriosis?
- If so, was it superficial or deep infiltrating?
- Where was it located and what stage would you consider it to be?
- Were you able to remove it all and how was this done? Ablation/excision—why/why not?
- Was there any damage to any of my organs?
- Were there adhesions and scar tissue?
- How is everything looking fertility-wise?

- Was there a suggestion of any other condition like adenomyosis? (Adenomyosis is like endo's evil sibling—more on this in Chapter 4.)
- What post-op symptoms or pain should I call you about or present myself to ER for (for example, infections, clots)?
- What are the next steps that you recommend for managing and treating my endo (for example, pelvic physio)?

Following your procedure, you should also be provided with:

- Post-op instructions specific to your situation (for example, when to get stitches out, when you can drive, exercise, lift/carry objects, have sexual intercourse, etc)
- Medical certificate for work/study.

The below may not be available until your first post-op appointment but it is important to request:

- Operation notes detailing what was detected, examined and removed
- Pathology results
- High-quality operation photographs of your endometriosis.

You are 1000 per cent entitled to these documents for your own health records. Plus, being your own health advocate means you need to be ready to pull out those receipts if something goes wrong or if you start seeing another specialist. Make sure you get them!

Another thing that will be occupying your mind is the next step in terms of recovery. How long will it take for things to feel normal again? When will the pain subside? The one thing about recovery that I can't stress enough is that it is different for everyone. This is due to a number of reasons, such as duration of procedure, extent of the endo found and removed, the doctor's surgical skills, how we respond to pain, additional conditions and more. No two people will have the same recovery, nor can you expect to have the same experience for each surgery.

To give you an idea, here are just some of the ways in which my two recoveries have differed:

2018

- Stayed overnight in hospital
- Vomited
- Painful bowel and bladder movements for at least a week
- Shoulder-tip pain from the carbon dioxide gas rising from my abdomen
- Instant period for nearly two weeks
- Took two weeks off work.

2020

- Stayed two nights in hospital with a drainage tube and catheter
- No vom!
- No shoulder-tip pain or painful bladder/bowel movements
- Nerve pain surrounding incision sites and neuropraxia in my upper thighs

- Bled for a few days and experienced first period two and a half weeks later
- Took four weeks off work.

You would think that recovery round two would have been easier, I certainly thought it would be! In many aspects, it was better but looking at it from a time-off-work perspective, things took a bit longer. Recovery is an overwhelming thing and you can never pre-determine how it will play out, so if I could share any tips with you, it would be these:

Accept that recovery is not linear

The road to recovery is not straight, my friend. She is windy, she is bumpy and she might be longer than you expect. You are going to experience some awesome days and you deserve to celebrate them but don't you dare beat yourself up on the shitty days. They're gonna happen but they're not going to erase the time and effort you have put into healing so far.

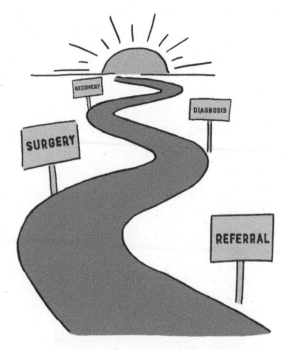

Listen to your body

This is so important. Only you know your true limits and if you don't listen to your body, you could end up doing more harm in the long run. I'll give you an example from my second surgery. I returned to work nineteen days after my procedure and I thought that was PLENTY of time, despite not feeling 100 per cent. I thought if I got my body back into the swing of things, she would adjust. I was oh-so wrong. I knew I was in for a difficult night the moment I arrived at my heavy, soundproof studio door. *Ah shit, I forgot about you.* With no-one else around, I struggled to do the most basic tasks, like opening that damn door, reaching across the panel to press buttons and make phone calls. I couldn't even bend down to adjust the chair! Two hours into my show and I could finally switch my microphone off and hit play on some pre-recorded live music sets. My fake smile quickly evaporated as I slumped on to the desk and burst into tears. It was a terribly painful shift but what I struggled most with was accepting that I wasn't ready to be at work again. So, I listened to my body and took the rest of the week off to continue my recovery. The following Monday, I was back on air, feeling *so* much better. All I needed was those extra few days.

Honour your feelings

Post-op blues are a real thing, y'all. They can be a reaction to a number of things, from the general anaesthetic and pain/discomfort to the lack of mobility and independence as you recover. With an invasive procedure like endometriosis surgery, we tend to just focus of the physical side, but your emotional state also needs to heal.

Even if your physical recovery is going really well, it's not unusual to become sensitive, anxious or agitated. You might even experience nightmares or randomly burst out sobbing and that is okay. I cannot begin to tell you how many times I ugly-cried into my heat pack, weeks after my surgery. Just remember that it will pass in time, so be gentle and patient with yourself. You got this!

During those overwhelming moments, try to make peace with what you cannot control (easier said than done, I know). Journal your feelings alongside your recovery progress and remember that every emotion is an experience you can learn from. You are doing your best.

This has been a pretty general overview of the surgical and healing process for removing endometriosis so keep in mind that every case is unique, but I hope you found it somewhat useful!

And while we're on the topic, I just want to put it out there and say that I think it is such BS that endometriosis surgery is generally treated as a day procedure, especially here in Australia and particularly through the public health system. I cannot disagree more with classifying this as a minor operation because it is Absolutely Not! We are talking about a procedure that can be so invasive and involves so many important organs. It affects your entire core and the recovery should not be downplayed. Not one bit. I've heard from many people who were discharged on the same day only to find themselves back in ER with a complication that prob-ably could have been avoided had they stayed overnight. Endometriosis surgery is not some in-and-out process like a fast food drive-thru. Dr Jeff Arrington recently said online, 'This disease is by far the most difficult surgical treatment we see in benign gynaecology. This is often a worse disease and more difficult surgery than gynaecological cancer.' If this is the case, then all healthcare systems need to reassess how endometriosis surgeries are dealt with in hospitals.

"

You are never alone in this experience. Don't let your mind convince you otherwise.

"

STEPHANIE CHINN

4

Associated conditions

Hey, well done you on making it this far! We've smashed through some solid information on endo and your brain probably feels like it's ready to explode, which is fair enough. Getting to know the basics of this complex disease is a pretty overwhelming process but look at you, ya bloody did it! I'm proud as punch.

Now, are you ready to meet the family?

... *Family?*

Hmm, yes, I *may* have failed to mention that endo has a bit of a crew. Sometimes it's just endo hanging out but you might catch it mingling with others. Distant relatives, you could say. But don't be nervous! I mean, I can't say they are harmless as these associated conditions aren't exactly a walk in the park, but I reckon they'll appreciate the fact that you've made some effort in getting to know who they are. You may never have to personally deal with these conditions but they're handy to be across, as learning about them can help broaden your understanding of endo and what your body is going through.

Adenomyosis

Say hi to adenomyosis! It's pretty much like endo's cousin and, between you and me, it's a piece of work too. Adeno is when the glands and stroma that comprise the endometrium (lining of the uterus) grow *within* the myometrium (muscle wall of the uterus).

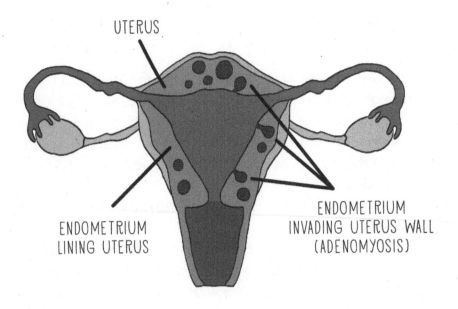

UTERUS

ENDOMETRIUM
LINING UTERUS

ENDOMETRIUM
INVADING UTERUS WALL
(ADENOMYOSIS)

Diagram of adenomyosis

The term is derived from the words:

- adeno—gland
- myo—muscle
- osis—condition.

Adenomyosis can be classified into two different patho-logic types:

→ **Diffuse adenomyosis**—this means more widespread. There is a diffuse non-capsulated involvement of both anterior and posterior walls of the uterus. The poste-rior wall is the most commonly affected side. Diffuse adenomyosis is found in approximately two-thirds of cases.

→ **Focal adenomyosis**—this means more nodular or local-ised to one area and results in an asymmetric uterus. The area of adenomyosis may have a pseudo-capsule, which is a structure, similar to a capsule, that surrounds some abnormal cells. Focal adenomyosis is found in one-third of cases.

Similar to endo, the cause of adenomyosis is unknown. There are a few theories floating around but nothing has been proven in clinical trials. Some people have both endo and adeno but having one doesn't mean you will necessarily have the other, despite some symptoms overlapping. Adeno symptoms may include:

- abnormal and/or heavy menstrual bleeding including blood clots
- lower back pain

- chronic pelvic pain
- painful sex
- painful bowel movements
- infertility
- upper thigh pain
- hip pain.

Another key sign of adeno is a soft, 'boggy', enlarged uterus. It is also worth noting that some people with adenomyosis are asymptomatic.

Like endo, adenomyosis isn't the easiest thing to diagnose. There are a few ways in which it may be detected such as:

→ **Manual pelvic examination**—which may reveal an enlarged and tender uterus.

→ **Expert guided transvaginal ultrasound (ETVUS)**—this involves a probe being placed in the vagina like a routine test. However, this one should preferably be performed by a gynaecologist who specialises in ultrasounds, as opposed to a general sonographer who may lack experience in diagnosing and detecting adenomyosis.

→ **MRI (magnetic resonance imaging)**—this collects pictures of soft tissue such as organs and muscles that don't show up on X-ray examinations.

The only true form of diagnosis is via pathology after a hysterectomy. That's right, while a hysterectomy cannot cure endo, it CAN diagnose and serve as a cure for adenomyosis because by removing the uterus, you are removing the adeno. Endo grows *outside* of the uterus, so taking the uterus out isn't going to stop the growth. Having a hysterectomy is not a decision to be made lightly, so please take time to consider the potential risks, complications and what's going to work best for you and your own situation. Your body, your choice.

In terms of pain management, there are a few options such as anti-inflammatory medications and hormonal treatments to alleviate symptoms but, again, they won't cure adeno. There are some instances where people with adenomyosis receive uterine ablation. This isn't the same as ablating endometriosis which is inferior to excision surgery. Uterine ablation involves burning of the endometrium to stop heavy bleeding, but this is not a permanent fix and it should not be performed if you intend to have children. There's also a procedure called a Presacral Neurectomy (PN) that surgically removes the presacral plexus, aka the group of nerves that conduct the pain signal from the uterus to the brain. It can be done via laparoscopy but it's a very delicate procedure with some risks, so you need to make sure you are dealing with a super-experienced specialist. Always consult with an informed medical professional.

Polycystic Ovary Syndrome (PCOS)

Next up, Polycystic Ovary Syndrome (PCOS). PCOS is a common but complex hormonal condition with its name referring to many cysts. The reason why it is labelled as a syndrome is because it involves a group of symptoms that affect the ovaries and ovulation. People with PCOS tend to have many partially formed follicles on the ovaries, which each contain an egg but these rarely reach maturity or trigger ovulation. The lack of ovulation alters levels of estrogen, progesterone, follicle stimulating hormone (FSH),

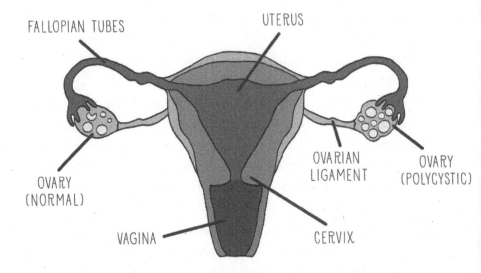

FALLOPIAN TUBES

UTERUS

OVARIAN LIGAMENT

OVARY (POLYCYSTIC)

OVARY (NORMAL)

VAGINA

CERVIX

Diagram of Polycystic Ovary Syndrome (PCOS)

and luteinising hormone (LH). Estrogen and progesterone levels are lower than usual, while androgen (male hormone) levels are higher than usual. Consequently, the menstrual cycle is disrupted, so those with PCOS get fewer periods.

Although some people may develop cysts on their ovaries, many do not. People with PCOS can also experience:

- weight gain
- fatigue
- unwanted hair growth (also known as hirsutism)
- thinning hair on the head
- infertility
- acne
- mood changes
- pelvic pain
- headaches

- sleep problems
- irregular periods
- increased inflammation in the body.

As you can see, some of the symptoms do overlap with endo so it is possible to have both but just because you have one doesn't necessarily mean you will have the other. To be diagnosed with PCOS, two of these three things must be present:

1. **Irregular/delayed periods**—or fancily referred to in the medical world as oligomenorrhea and anovulation
2. **Hyperandrogenism**—we're talking characteristics such as acne, scalp hair loss or increased facial and/or body hair growth, or a blood test showing higher levels of androgen hormones
3. **Twenty follicles on either ovary**—detected via ultrasound.

The list above is known as the Rotterdam Criteria, formed in 2003 to help health professionals correctly diagnose PCOS. A long-term approach is key to managing PCOS as there is no cure but treatment options such as diet and lifestyle changes and birth control should all be discussed with a medical professional.

The four Ds

The four Ds aren't the easiest to pronounce but they're pretty straightforward. Many medical professionals are very familiar with these conditions and will usually point to them before an endometriosis diagnosis.

Dysmenorrhoea (dis-meh-nuh-ree-ah)

This is the medical term for excessive pain when menstruating. There are two types of dysmenorrhoea. Primary dysmenorrhoea typically occurs in the absence of pelvic disease. Secondary dysmenorrhoea results from anatomic or macroscopic pelvic pathology, as seen in people with endometriosis or chronic pelvic inflammatory disease. So, if your medical professional ever mentions secondary, they definitely need to be exploring further for endo.

Dysuria (dis-ur-ria)

This condition is characterised by pain or discomfort when urinating. Your doctor can usually make a diagnosis based on symptoms you describe and the analysis of a urine sample (urinalysis). Treatment for dysuria can vary from prescribed medication to eliminating chemicals from shower gels and body lotions, but it really depends on the cause of the pain, whether it's due to infection, inflammation, dietary factors, or a problem with the bladder.

Dyschezia (dis-keez-ia)

Dyschezia involves excessive straining with stools. It's basically lacking coordination within the pelvic muscles when pooping and while it is often seen in babies and toddlers, dyschezia can also affect adults. Exercises for the pelvic floor are usually recommended to help as well as diet modifications.

Dyspareunia (dis-par-roo-nea)

This condition presents as pain as a result of penetrative sexual intercourse or activity. It can be diagnosed based on medical and sexual history and via a manual pelvic exam. If your doctor suspects a particular cause for dyspareunia (that is, endo), they may refer you for an ultrasound. Some ways this condition can be treated are through pelvic physiotherapy and seeing a sexologist.

Dyspareunia can often be mistaken for two other conditions: vulvodynia and vaginismus. Vulvodynia is chronic pain or discomfort around the opening of your vagina (vulva), whereas vaginismus occurs when the muscles around the vagina tighten or spasm involuntarily. Vaginismus usually occurs when the genital area is touched but it's not just about sexytime. This pain may occur before attempting to insert a tampon or during a gynaecological examination.

Fibromyalgia

Fibromyalgia is a chronic and complex condition that involves widespread, ongoing pain affecting various systems in the body. It is not considered an autoimmune or inflammation-based illness but, according to the American College of Rheumatology, research suggests the nervous system is involved. Because of its multi-system nature, it's common for people to experience different symptoms but the most common include:

- pain and tenderness in joints and muscles
- fatigue, lack of energy and trouble sleeping.

Fibro can be fierce, man. I have friends with the condition who experience sensitivity to wearing clothing or even to light. The severity and debilitating nature of some of the symptoms were echoed in a US National Health Interview Survey: 87 per cent of participants reported having pain on most days or every day of their lives. There is no set test for fibromyalgia so it can be quite difficult to diagnose as your doctor must solely rely on your reporting of your symptoms. Medications, cognitive behavioural therapies and gentle exercise may assist in the management of fibro but there is no cure.

Irritable Bowel Syndrome (IBS)

Have you ever been mistaken for somebody else? In high school, I was frequently told that I looked like another girl in Ballarat and I vividly remember meeting my alleged doppelganger while working at McDonald's one night. The restaurant was full and I was serving at the front counter when, among the crowd of customers, Elle appeared at my register. It was so amusing as we stared at each other with wide eyes and big smiles, knowing exactly who the other was. We laughed as we could finally see why so many people told us how similar we looked. I resembled Elle more than my actual biological twin! (Yes, I am a twin.)

I feel like endo and IBS would have a similar reaction if they ever ran into each other because it is SO common to be diagnosed with IBS instead of endometriosis. They're like distant cousins who on first glance look more like siblings, but as you get to know them you see how they differ. There is no medical test to detect IBS—rather, it is usually based on reported symptoms and medical history. Therefore, it can be pretty easy and convenient for medical professionals to suggest this condition instead of considering the fact that endometriosis may actually be present on the bowel or somewhere on the gastrointestinal tract.

Irritable Bowel Syndrome is pretty self-explanatory—a condition affecting the functioning of the bowel. The main symptoms of IBS include:

- recurring diarrhoea or constipation
- bloating
- pain or discomfort that is relieved by passing wind or going to the toilet.

IBS can be managed in numerous ways. One is through modification of diet (specifically increasing fibre and eliminating triggers). Another may be stress management as stress may influence IBS flare-ups. Some people may require medical therapy and, in extreme cases, surgical intervention for complications like bowel obstruction (blockage) or abscesses (built up pus). Pelvic physiotherapy can also help, which you will learn more about later in this book.

Interstitial Cystitis (IC)

Trying saying this one fast! IC is a chronic pelvic pain issue that is basically the sibling of IBS but, instead of bowel issues, we're looking at irritative bladder symptoms. These can include:

- a persistent, urgent need to urinate
- pain in pelvis or between the vagina and anus
- frequent urination, often small amounts, throughout the day and night

- pain/discomfort while the bladder fills and relief after urinating
- painful sexual intercourse.

In terms of diagnosis, there are a few options. Alongside reported symptoms and a manual pelvic exam, a urinalysis may be required as well as a cystoscopy. During this procedure, a tube-like instrument called a cystoscope is inserted through your urethra and into your bladder to detect ulcers, swelling and any possible signs of infection. During this procedure, a biopsy may be taken from the bladder and the urethra to check for bladder cancer and other rare causes of bladder pain.

Treating interstitial cystitis may require a multimodal approach through means of pelvic physio, oral medications and the use of a TENS machine which may increase blood flow to the bladder.

Uterine fibroids

Finally, meet fibroids. Also known as a myoma, fibroids are non-cancerous tumours that grow in and around the uterus. Like many of these associated conditions, the cause of fibroids is unknown and while it is common to be asymptomatic, some symptoms are similar to endometriosis:

- heavy and/or prolonged menstrual bleeding
- pelvic pressure/pain
- frequent urination and/or difficulty emptying the bladder
- constipation
- backache or leg pains.

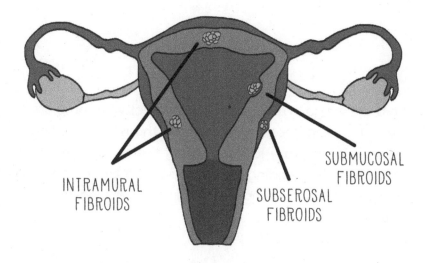

Diagram of uterine fibroids

There are three major types of uterine fibroids:

1. **Intramural fibroids**—found within the muscular uterine wall
2. **Submucosal fibroids**—found more towards the uterine cavity
3. **Subserosal fibroids**—found closer to the outside of the uterus.

They can be detected via gynaecological examination, pelvic ultrasound or during surgical procedures such as hysteroscopy or laparoscopy, usually intended for other conditions. Treatment options for fibroids are super varied depending on their size, number and location, and range from just monitoring them to taking medication or undergoing a surgical procedure to remove them. It's best to consult with your specialist.

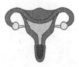

So there we go, a quick little meet'n'greet with some associates of endometriosis. Keep in mind, though, that all of this information is really just scratching the surface so I highly recommend extending your research on these conditions and, as always, speaking to a medical professional for further clarification.

how to deal

You know you have endo when . . .

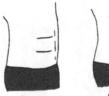
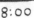
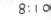

→ You have abs at 8 a.m. and look five months pregnant by 8:10 a.m.

→ Jeans do not exist in your vocabulary, let alone your wardrobe.

→ White pants? I simply do not know her.

→ You see your specialists more than your friends.

→ You start talking to your heat pack. You also pat it like a treasured pet. *Goooood girl!*

→ 5/10 is a successful pain day. WOO!

→ What cramps? All I feel is the burning of my skin from my heat pack! This is fine!

→ Your purse is actually a pop-up pharmacy that could cater for your entire suburb.

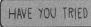

→ The only action in your DMs is from people asking 'Have you tried . . . ?'

→ You buy your clothes in two sizes—one for normal wear, one for bloating and flare-ups.

5

Social media and
self-advocacy

Okay, I'm about to spill some piping hot tea on you, much like the time I literally fell asleep sitting upright in bed with a cup of piping hot tea in my hand. I'm still trying to get the stains out of my doona. ANYWAY, here we go . . .

I have learned more about my endometriosis from social media than from any consultation with any medical professional. Yep. I know that sounds bizarre, and it IS bizarre, but that is the (kinda sad) reality for anyone suffering an invisible, incurable condition like endo. The lack of awareness, support and education from the medical field has given sufferers no choice but to be their own advocates AND their own experts.

Upon my diagnosis, endometriosis was just a name for my pain but it wasn't until I chose to embark on a journey of self-advocacy and education that I came to know the true depths of this chronic disease and the ways in which it had already influenced my life and what it meant for me moving forward.

How does it make you feel reading that? Scared that you're not qualified enough to self-advocate? Confused because as a sufferer, that shouldn't even be your role anyway? I FEEL YOU. Now, I'm *definitely* not saying that we should dismiss our doctors' advice, pretty pls do not do that! But the unfortunate fact of the matter is that much of their advice is simply *not enough* and will not equip us with the adequate information we truly need to navigate life with endometriosis. Therefore, we need to take it upon ourselves to find the missing pieces of our endo puzzle. And just like we do for many other things—recipes, reviews, even the weather—we turn to the internet.

According to Google Health boss David Feinberg, the popular search engine receives approximately 70,000 health-related searches every minute. That figure does not surprise me, but I wonder how often people really find the answer they are looking for. And when it comes to an isolating, misunderstood condition like endometriosis, sufferers are searching for more than answers. They are searching for *validation* and *comfort*. Not only do we feel neglected by the medical system, but we can also feel hugely isolated from our friends and family. God love 'em, but sometimes they just really don't get it. This is where social media enters the chat (cue old-school MSN Messenger notification sound, am I showing my age here?).

These days, it's pretty easy to associate social media with influencers and fake news (cheers, Trump). But I'm here to guide you past the teeth-whitener #sponcon and general misinformation to help you find what you *really* need. Before

I share some tips on using social media for your endo, I'd love to take you through my own experience.

My endo social life began on Facebook after booking in for my first surgery in 2018. My friend Hayleigh put me on to one local support group and from there, I joined a few others to seek as much advice as possible regarding surgery prep and recovery. I didn't really have any expectations, but I found sooo much comfort in these online communities. Not only was I surrounded by people who actually understood what I was going through and how I was feeling but I knew they were there, willing and ready to pass on what they had learned from their own experiences. If it wasn't for these groups, I would have never known that there are two ways to surgically remove endo and which is the superior method. Nor the true wonders of peppermint tea in relieving the post-surgery gas pain from your shoulder tips. About the importance of requesting your operation notes and photos for your own records. To meal prep because cooking after surgery is the LAST thing you'll wanna do. Things that were never covered in my appointments or in the brochures I received, but were essential to my endo journey. I also probably would not have found my current specialist either!

After sharing my diagnosis on triple j, I received countless DMs from listeners with endo, as well as those who thought they might have it. I even got messages from their friends/partners who wanted to learn more about the condition! My heart! Whenever I'd do a Q&A on Instagram, I would always be asked how I was recovering or what advice I could pass on, so in May 2019, I launched endogram. A separate account to my personal page, I wanted endogram to have a ~strong aesthetic~. Or, in my language, I wanted it to be a fucking FABULOUS visual delight—full of vibrant illustrations and work from contemporary artists with informative captions exploring different aspects of this chronic illness. I always wanted endogram to be particularly accessible for a younger audience because I can *totally* empathise with how difficult it is to have these kinds of conversations with your peers and the fear of being judged for your pain. In high school, I wasn't taught a damn thing about endo and if I had been, I reckon it could have drastically decreased the time it took for me to get an official diagnosis. Instead of twelve years from first experiencing symptoms, it could have been two years. I'll never forget receiving a message from a sixteen-year-old who told me how much endogram has helped her start conversations with her friends in school because they all love the artwork I share. THAT is what it's about, fam!

I seriously love Instagram. It's my favourite social media platform and a large majority of my daily screen time is aaaabsolutely thanks to my relentless scrolling on it. Yeah, there's a bit of rubbish and filtered perceptions of life that may be a bit eyeroll-y but let me tell you, Instagram has been my main gateway to a powerful and passionate community of endometriosis advocates. From celebrities like Alexa Chung, Sarah Hyland and Lena Dunham to people just like you and me, it's crazy how a few hashtags can lead to an incredible network of people who stand in solidarity, despite living thousands of kilometres apart. Through endogram, I have forged genuine friendships with people that I've never even met. I am constantly inspired by the validating posts of Georgia Stuart (@theendojournal) who reminds me it's okay to slow down and listen to my body. And the no-bullshit approach of Kellie Niebling (@thatendogoddess) who will fearlessly shut down any insincere marketing scheme or fear-mongering content directed at our already vulnerable patient community.

One of my closest connections is with Claudia Wright (a.k.a. @me_myself_and_endometriosis), who shares the ups and downs of living with multiple chronic conditions with over 9000 followers. Claudia, who launched her account in 2018 about five months following her diagnosis, says this about it:

> My health was rapidly declining, I was six weeks away from flying to the US for surgery, expecting my period and had just been discharged from the hospital after an accidental overdose trying to control my severe pain.
>
> The account was made almost immediately after returning home. I didn't even think about the name for more than ten minutes, I just knew I wanted to scream about how serious endometriosis is!

Like me, Claudia quickly realised the power and potential of social media to help people with chronic conditions.

> In the months following my diagnostic surgery and leading up to starting this account, I was researching everything I could about endo. I quickly became blown away because the most factual, evidence-based data I could find was on social media, presented by those who had fought through hell with this disease, made it out and then were kind enough to come back with supplies for those of us still struggling. Reading this information and hearing these stories truly changed my life in a number of ways. It taught me the facts of this disease, how it should be treated and who could treat it. It introduced me to friends I will have for life. It made

me feel validated and part of a community. But it also ignited a type of burning passion inside, like nothing I had experienced before.

To put it simply, Claudia knows her shit. From her posts and story highlights to endless Q&A sessions, Claudia puts an immense amount of time into creating her content and ensuring that it is accurate and accessible. She even launched a gorgeous endo necklace for people to purchase online and it sold out worldwide, within minutes! Beyond endo, we have also found similarities in the music we enjoy, our shared outlook on life—and it turns out we even share the same birthday. We are literally endo-sisters, just a few hours apart! To think that I found her and my own online support system simply by punching a few endo hashtags into my Instagram search bar is pretty damn cool.

The great news is that you and I can share the same social media outcomes. You are SO WELCOME to tap into this empowering endometriosis community, share your story and form friendships with those who are going through the same struggles. The (Instagram) world is your oyster!

Not gonna lie though, getting started can be a bit over-whelming. Like, where do you begin? All it can take is one hashtag to lead you into an overflowing feed of content from bloated endo bellies to fertility updates, post-surgical scars and even crying selfies which is totally fine but it can be a bit triggering at times. You may feel like you are suddenly taking on an extra emotional load as you expose yourself to other people's experiences. Or it may instead bring you a great deal of comfort—we all react differently and that is absolutely okay.

Here are some tips that I hope will help you make the most of endo social media. ♡

Establish your purpose—what are you really looking for?

Everyone is on endo social media for different reasons. You may want to make new friends, feel less alone or you might just want to find some specific information regarding endometriosis. You are in control of your intent and what you consume, so it's important to stop and ask yourself: 'What do I want to get to out of this?' Knowing the answer to that question will help you navigate the Explore feed and the accounts you choose to follow and connect with.

If you are there purely to seek accurate information, I would recommend joining Nancy's Nook Endometriosis Education. Just type those four words into your Facebook search bar and you will come across a private group with over 100,000 members. Yep, that's how popular it's become. The group primarily consists of patients but there are also loved ones and even a bunch of doctors and endometriosis specialists who are members. This group is described as a self-serve library. There's no open discussions that provide support as such, instead members are encouraged to use the files to find the info they need and become their own expert. It's factual and frank.

If you're looking for support groups where you can have a vent and a D&M with other endo warriors, best to look elsewhere. Find out if your national organisation runs any online support groups, for example QENDO (Australia) has Facebook groups for all capital cities. They also organise Endo Meets—whether that is in person or via Zoom—offering a safe space for you to share your problems. It's a cost-effective way of connecting with new people and, heck, these interactions could even save you from splashing coin on a therapy session!

Put yourself out there—you can do it!

This one applies to anyone who wants to make a post, create an endo account or reach out to a fellow warrior for advice or friendship. For one of my endogram giveaways, I wanted my followers to share their most recent endo win. Something that they were really proud of and wanted to celebrate or acknowledge. The responses were all so amazing but I was particularly proud to hear from those who decided to open up and share their own journey with others.

> I posted on Instagram about my endo experience so far and was able to help a few girls after they reached out about their own personal concerns. I was nervous to post but realised I needed to raise awareness and try and help others—@elishadalli

If it's any comfort, I was totally shitting myself about creating endogram. I was so scared of judgement. I was worried it would be received poorly but I put myself out there and it's pretty much led me to writing this book! It is always a daunting thing to step out of your comfort zone and use your voice, but you deserve to be heard and your story is so important to share! Never forget that. Plus, you can make some seriously awesome connections with people all around the world.

Just because endo accounts are run by endo patients does not mean they can or should give you medical advice

Okay, this one is really important, fam. There's a difference between learning about endo on social media and taking medical advice about endo on social media. Big difference.

Unless someone can legitimately prove they are qualified, they cannot and should not be handing out such sensitive information. Nopeeee, nope, nope. It's super irresponsible and can do more harm than good. Endometriosis is already complex enough as it is, we don't want to be making it even more complicated. Plus, we all deal with the condition and its symptoms SO differently. My experience with pain and particular treatments may not be the same for you and vice versa. Whether it's concerning birth control, hysterectomies, which specialist to see—use the information you obtain from social media to make informed decisions for yourself.

I'm all about providing factual information regarding these things—for example, hysterectomies cannot cure endometriosis. But nobody can say, 'YOU should/should not do this' because they simply don't know your situation. Your body, your choice. Plus, if you're not sure about something that has been posted, ask for further details like a website or study, or you can consult a credible source like Nancy's Nook or the Center for Endometriosis Care. It's pretty easy for false information to spread like wildfire, so always ensure what you are sharing and what you are consuming is factual.

Beware of people trying to use your condition to sell you stuff!!!

We know the internet can be pretty dodgy and, unfortunately, vulnerable people with chronic illness make for easy targets when it comes to money-making. Let's start with MLM. If you're not across it, MLM is short for Multi-Level Marketing, and is also referred to as network/referral marketing or word of mouth/direct/pyramid selling. Products and services are sold but distributors associated with the company can also earn income by recruiting new sellers—so for each sale their 'down line' makes, the referring distributor earns a small commission. This can be done through DM transactions (buying via your social media inboxes) or promoting through private groups . . . that kind of thing.

MLM strategy has drawn criticism for having a similar business model to that of a pyramid scheme. It's a complex conversation for our community in particular, because from a sales perspective, it could actually be a perfect job for a chronic-illness sufferer. Flexible hours, work from home, your own client base—you're essentially the boss of your own small business. It kinda reminds me of when I was a travel agent, as your desk was referred to as your own business. We were responsible for what sales and commission we made.

Now, I appreciate the hustle, but I have a huuuge problem with strategies like MLM deciding to target people who they know are so desperate for relief that they are willing to try anything. People like you and me. These strategies use our vulnerability and suffering to their advantage by selling products not on the basis of evidence but on emotion. They not only use our condition as a buzzword and a selling point, but they are often unqualified to be peddling products that are labelled as health and wellness. It's gross and there's a reason why these strategies are banned from multiple groups that are moderated by legitimate endo organisations.

My mate Kellie has had her fair share of people sliding into her DMs and inviting her to private 'wellness' groups that are full of products directed at endo and PCOS sufferers. She shared on her Instagram:

> I used to be that vulnerable young girl wasting all my money on products because another girl on the internet said it worked for her. So many of these multi-level marketers don't care about their audience. You're talking about a disease that at times destroys mental health, impacts relationships and can potentially shatter people's chances of becoming parents. It's not a fucking fad to make fast cash.

Like Kellie, I was invited to join a private Facebook group to learn more about some oral drops for endo. I was hugely sceptical—particularly because the single PDF product description that I was provided with made no mention of endometriosis—but I was still curious about the testimonials that alleged these drops could eliminate endo symptoms. As I scrolled through the posts, I found two common themes—weight loss and the number of surgeries that people had for their endo. We're talking ten or more surgeries, which is really concerning. For one person to have that many surgeries suggests a few things—the use of ablation, the continuous formation of adhesions as a result of ablation and a regular OB-GYN who is not equipped to deal with endometriosis. Instead, the focus of the posts was on how these drops saved them and did a better job than any surgery could. These posts were riding on emotion and not facts, so I wanted to help and share some additional information and evidence-based tips. My post was deleted by admins because 'it didn't fit with what the page is about and what the hub provides'. I was removed from the group shortly after.

So, look, you are free to try whatever you want, but if you ever receive an unsolicited message about a product claiming to heal your endo, be super cautious. Oral drops, powdered drinks, vaginal steaming, supplements and even CBD come up on these posts. The most effective thing you can do for your endo is to get it excised.

Alongside MLM, be wary of 'coaches'. I'm talking life coaches, wellbeing coaches, even 'endo coaches'. Not only is coaching an unregulated industry—anyone can claim to be one—but nothing actually defines their scope of practice. Whilst we may be the experts of our own bodies, having endometriosis does not qualify anyone to coach or manage another person's illness, especially if they're offering to do this purely online. If you want to seek expert advice for managing your endo, please make sure you check the qualifications and credentials of the people who claim that they can help you.

Language matters

I try to be very careful with how I talk about endometriosis because it doesn't just affect women. As you will read later in the book, there are also transgender and non-binary people who suffer from this condition and our language can really influence how they navigate the health system. Constantly referring to endo as a 'women's health condition' is not inclusive. Endo is already isolating enough as it is, let's not make it even harder for our fellow trans and non-binary warriors. ♡

Check in with yourself

This is so important because, as I mentioned earlier, by exposing yourself to the endo experiences of others, you may subconsciously be taking on an extra emotional load and that may not be so great for you. Even sharing your own story can be quite draining. Make sure you monitor your social media usage and especially stay aware of how everything is making you *feel*. Do you feel better from seeing this content or is it making things worse for you? If it's helping, great! If it's not, it's time to reassess what you are consuming, who it's from and how to change it. It's also important to maintain that balance of online community and physical connection with the people around you. Like the sixteen-year-old girl I mentioned at the start of this chapter, how cool that she could show her friends my posts which sparked face-to-face conversation and understanding? It's important that we take breaks and that we don't entirely shut off from the people physically around us. It's not healthy to consume social media all the time about a condition that already takes up so much of your physical energy. Look after yourself!

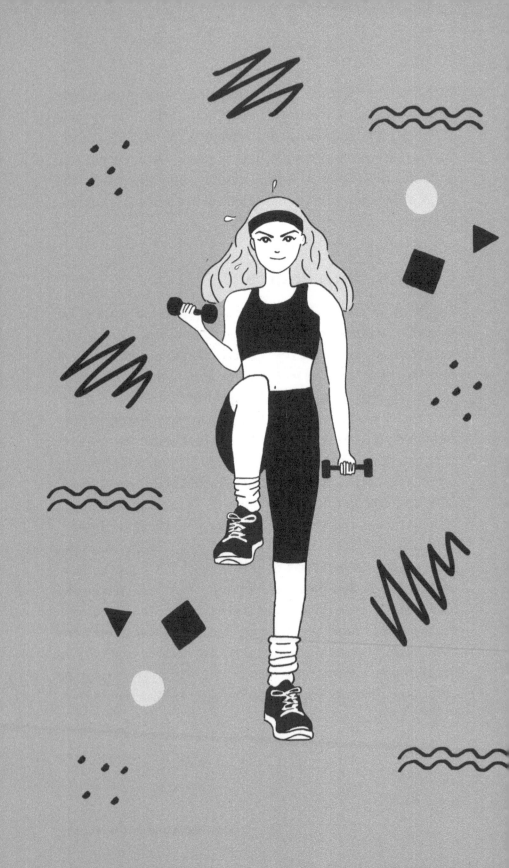

6

Let's get physical (therapy)

As we know, the average time it takes for someone to be diagnosed with endometriosis is six and a half years. That, my friend, is a LONG time to not only obtain answers, but it's also plenty of time for endo to cause some real havoc inside. From nerve hypersensitivity and muscle spasms to postural alignment problems and a weakened core, a lengthy diagnosis can result in *years* of damage for many people and, unfortunately, that cannot be resolved by surgery alone.

Taking the disease out at its root through excision is, of course, the gold standard but a common misconception is that it will also remove our symptoms. I wish it were that easy! In order to fully get on top of our endo management, we need to take a multidisciplinary approach.

A multi-huh?

Sounds a bit fancy, right? A multidisciplinary approach essentially means combining specialities and looking at endo from a whole-body perspective because, let's be real, it *is* a whole-body disease. There's such a wide varying range of symptoms but when you think about it, endo has a real domino effect on our bodies. Pain can rear up in so many different areas and it can be triggered by various things such as diet and sex. Pain can also affect our mental health and our relationships. We owe it to ourselves to address all of these things and the most effective way of doing so is through the formation of a multidisciplinary team.

More specialists = more money?

Unfortunately, yeah, bringing more people on board means working out that bank account. Endometriosis is *expensive*. As tax time was nearing, I thought it would be fun (?) to look through my bank statements and calculate my out-of-pocket expenses for endometriosis in the last twelve months (1 July 2019–1 July 2020).

- Acupuncture and traditional Chinese medicine (TCM)—$1559
- Pelvic physio—$1192
- Specialist appointments—$400
- Ultrasounds—$350
- Private health insurance—$1658
- Surgery (surgeon out-of-pocket gap fee, anaesthetist out-of-pocket, hospital fee, insurance excess $200)—$6150
- Total = $11,309

For a visual representation of my reaction to this total, please google 'Kristen Bell Laugh Cry GIF'.

I then did what none of us should do and pondered what that money could have gone towards. A (pre-COVID) holiday, a decent second-hand car, a little juice-up to my house savings . . . It was like self-inflicted salt in the wound.

Although I had to implement some budgeting in order to afford these costs, I'm still privileged that I could make it work. It's just so utterly sad that as endometriosis sufferers, we have to go to such financial lengths in order to live a *semi-normal* life. I cannot help but feel for those who are unable to be in a similar position, because the extent of their endo does not allow them the comfort or stability to earn consistent streams of income.

In 2019, research from Western Sydney University and the University of New South Wales revealed that endometriosis costs an individual and society $30,000 per year. Around one-fifth of this cost was in the health sector, for medications, doctors' visits, hospital visits, assisted reproductive technology such as IVF and any transport costs to get to these appointments. Of this, $1200 were out-of-pocket costs.

It's pretty simple: our quality of life with endometriosis is dictated by money. But that's why I'm here as your wing-woman to not only navigate this condition, but the costs associated with it as well. I want to save you a few coins before you start calling everyone and anyone for appointments. Think of the next few chapters as speed dating. I'm going to give you a taste of each component and introduce you to some experts who will share some vital information to help you make the best decisions for your situation. It's then up to you to swipe left or right on the areas you think are important to focus on in your multidisciplinary approach to endometriosis.

For our first stop, let's get physical!

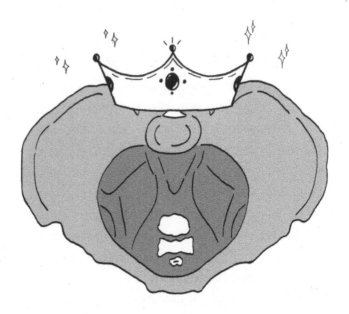

Your pelvic floor absolutely deserves a crown

The pelvic palace

Welcome to the pelvic floor, or as I like to call it, the pelvic palace! It's a group of muscles that are arranged within the pelvis, almost like a hammock, connecting the front, back, and sides of the pelvis and sacrum. The main purpose of these muscles is to provide support to the organs of the pelvis and allow normal urination, bowel movements and sexual intercourse.

I refer to it as a palace because I'll take any opportunity for alliteration but, also, I think it's a really important part of our body that we really should treat like royalty! Especially when we are dealing with endometriosis which can cause some pretty big dysfunctions. In fact, endometriosis has a strong association to Pelvic Floor Dysfunction (PFD), with abnormal muscle tension developing as a protective response to our pain. Pelvic Floor Dysfunction is when these muscles cannot effectively coordinate contraction and relaxation. Consequently, PFD can cause some or all of the following symptoms:

- urinary urgency, frequency, hesitancy, stopping and starting the stream of urine, painful urination, or inability to empty the bladder
- constipation, straining, pain with bowel movements
- lower back pain or pain in the pelvic region, genital area or rectum
- pain during or after intercourse, orgasm or sexual stimulation
- uncoordinated muscle contractions causing the pelvic floor muscles to spasm.

Think about all those bad periods that have caused you to crawl into a foetal position. While it's a basic protective response to pain, curling up in this position actually creates tension within your abdominal muscles, the inner thigh muscles and pelvic floor muscles. Similarly, if you feel pain during penetrative sex, a natural response is to squeeze the muscles around your vagina. That kinda stuff can't really be fixed by surgery. In order to address the dysfunction found in the muscles of the pelvic floor, we need to look at pelvic floor therapy. This can be done by seeing a physical therapist or physiotherapist who specialises in pelvic pain.

I personally was super hesitant to see a pelvic physio following my first surgery because everything I'd heard about it sounded pretty invasive. By everything, I mean the constant reference to kegel balls which, by the way, are not beneficial for people with endo so if you're ever told to use one, RUN! It also didn't help that the random bulk-billing GP I saw admitted they didn't know of any highly regarded therapists. Extremely comforting!

It wasn't until I returned to Melbourne in 2019 that I started seeking recommendations via endo support groups and found Alison Harding, a physiotherapist with a Graduate Certificate in Pelvic Floor and Women's Health. I left our first consultation feeling so relieved that I was in the hands of someone who practised in such an informative and caring manner. What I also love about my sessions is that I have gained a greater understanding of the pain process within my pelvic palace. Being aware of how the muscles work and respond makes me feel so much more in sync with my body and I find that really comforting. So, say hi to Ali! She has answered some questions to help you form a better understanding of her field.

What is the role of a physiotherapist and pelvic floor therapy in managing endometriosis?

Physiotherapists provide a whole-body approach to assessment and management of endometriosis. The journey will often start with taking a thorough history and listening to the person's story. As many who have experienced endo will know, this can be quite a long and winding road and an individual's story helps us, as physios, to develop a strong sense of possible contributing factors and a path in to start promoting new learning and change with our bodies and pain system. Pelvic floor physios will assess a number of systems within your body. This can involve your musculoskeletal system (muscles and bones/joints), your pain system (central nervous system), your whole nervous system, your bladder and bowel health, your sexual health and your exercise history.

When it comes to endometriosis, what can sometimes be overlooked is how our body and its protective pain system respond to the ongoing tissue changes that occur in the pelvis as a result of the condition. Our pain system is our warning or alert system, and we know sometimes in cases where people have experienced longer term pain, it can become sensitive and extra protective. This can result in the body misinterpreting general sensations as painful (for example, someone lightly touching your stomach or pelvis). What we also know is that our muscles, bones, joints, ligaments and nerves are very good at protecting us. When this becomes maladaptive, it can result in dysfunction in many muscles around the pelvis, including the abdominal muscles, your hip muscles, lower back muscles and certainly the internal pelvic floor muscles. Over time, these muscle groups can become tense and protective, leading to poor coordination and relaxation, in turn leading to a number of symptoms which can include issues with bladder and bowel emptying, painful intercourse and pelvic pain. This muscle tension can contribute to the pain experienced with periods.

By assessing any musculoskeletal changes and using a number of tools to evaluate the sensitivity of your pain system, we can start working together on treatment and self-management strategies. Many people are often surprised by the relief that can be achieved from treating these broader musculoskeletal issues and addressing your pain system changes. Physiotherapists are strong advocates of informed care and provide education to empower and promote self-management strategies, working with you and your other health professionals to provide a true, multidisciplinary team approach.

Whether you have had surgery, plan to have surgery or if surgery is not an option for you, assessing and treating your whole body will help aid recovery, prepare you for surgery, and in many cases can be an effective option to help you understand your pain, take back control and dramatically improve your quality of life.

Treatment usually involves a number of options and can include: resources to explain and understand your pain, manual therapy or hands-on treatment techniques to address any of the aforementioned findings, pelvic floor down-training or relaxation strategies, pelvic floor muscle release, dilators (or trainers)—which are used to desensitise the pelvic floor muscles to information they are receiving, bladder and bowel health education and advice on emptying and mechanics, sexual rehab specific strategies and general exercise and lifestyle advice. As this is a complex condition with many facets, not all of this will be relevant to every person with endo and everybody's starting point will be different!

How do I know if I need to see a physio and how would I go about finding the right person?

In my (perhaps biased!) opinion, almost all those with endometriosis could learn and benefit from seeing a pelvic health physiotherapist. It can be very empowering to learn about the connections within your own body and the relationship endo has with other structures in the body.

If you have experienced symptoms including pelvic pain, abdominal, lower back and hip pain, painful intercourse, vulval pain, bladder issues (including difficulty emptying, pain with emptying, frequency and urgency), bowel issues (difficulty emptying, constipation, pain with a bowel action, bloating and gut concerns) and difficulty engaging in your regular activities such as exercise and work, then it is likely that a pelvic floor physio would be able to help!

When it comes to choosing the right person as your physio, it is important to find someone who has experience in treating pelvic pain and, equally importantly, someone who fits well with you. Your therapist will form an integral part of your care team, therefore, it is crucial to find someone who you will be able to work well with so you feel confident that you are seeing progress with your treatment.

Often GPs, gynaecologists and other specialists will be able to refer you to someone within your local area. There are also a number of websites that list physiotherapists in your area with experience in pelvic health, including CFA Physios Victoria and the APA (Australian Physiotherapy Association). Some public hospitals have specialised pelvic pain clinics and the Jean Hailes Foundation also has a pelvic pain clinic with a multidisciplinary team, including physiotherapists. If you are part of any support groups, you will also often be able to find recommendations from other members.

At the end of the day, the most important thing is finding the right person for you. Someone to have in your corner and to form part of your team!

What does the first appointment typically involve?

The first appointment will start with taking a history and talking through your concerns. People may present to a physio at any stage, so it is important to gauge what their current goals are, in order to direct treatment. Pelvic floor physios understand that you are the most important person in your care team. We aim to work together, with you, to establish goals, suitable and reasonable treatment options, and support to allow you to improve your quality of life. By adopting this model of patient-centred care, we find we are able to individually tailor treatment options, promoting more successful outcomes. There is no one-size-fits-all approach when it comes to dealing with the wide world of endo.

A physical examination will usually occur over a number of sessions and can include: an analysis of your movement, including lower back, hips and pelvis, the quality and function of muscle groups within your body and often, at a time that is appropriate, a pelvic floor muscle examination, which is usually an internal vaginal examination. Care will be taken by the physio to ensure the examination is done in a timely manner for each person and you will be talked through each step of the process. These examinations help inform your treating therapist of the condition of your muscles in order to allow more targeted treatment and can also provide invaluable feedback about your own body—so you can again start to regain control and learn how to make the appropriate changes!

These assessments and examinations all help to develop a tailored treatment approach, which is the best way to achieve optimal outcomes. If you don't feel something is relevant to you, have this conversation with your physio! We are very good listeners and we know the best outcomes come from working together in a collaborative approach.

How frequent would visits need to be and when do people typically start to notice changes?

Everyone's path is different and we often describe the journey as one with small speed bumps along the way. However, a generalised treatment program would usually start with a series of approximately fortnightly appointments (taking into consideration a number of individual circumstances), for between three and twelve months, and then likely progress to monthly appointments and ongoing reviews as required. As with all things endo, the symptom spectrum is enormous and some may require far less physio, others may be involved with physio for longer, depending on the degree of contributing factors that can be addressed by physiotherapy.

What we often notice is that people experience small progressive changes and we would expect to see this from the beginning of our journey together. Our goal is to establish a new baseline within your body and build on that, with foundational and functional steps until we reach your goals. As you will be learning a lot about how different parts of your body work and interact, many people are amazed by the things they didn't know! It can be transformative and empowering to have a new-found awareness, confidence and understanding of your pelvis, and this will open the door to reclaiming this part of your body.

Endometriosis is a costly condition to manage. Do you have any tips for people who may not be able to afford regular consults or things we could do at home to support our pelvic floor?

One of the most beneficial things is to discuss with your GP the option of an Enhanced Primary Care Plan. While everyone may not be eligible, it can sometimes be an option for people and provides a Medicare rebate for a certain number of sessions, which is very helpful to ease some of the financial burden. We are also fortunate to have many excellent public health clinics and facilities in Australia that can be accessed through referral by your GP. There are many valuable resources on the internet, including Endometriosis Australia, Jean Hailes, EndoActive and guided pelvic floor relaxation videos/recordings, etc which can be a nice starting point for learning about your pelvis.

If you can be connected with a pelvic floor physio, they will often be able to tailor a treatment program to suit your constraints, where you can learn a lot and get started. It's amazing what a difference a session or two can make!

What forms of exercise would you consider to be endo-friendly?

Everyone is different and what works for one person may not be appropriate for the next. We are often recommending exercise routines that promote functional use of 'core' muscles—including abs, lower back and pelvic floor. For many people, gentle forms of yoga, encouraging lengthening, breathing, opening and stretching can be very useful. We also find many people with endo often respond well to low-impact exercise, which helps release happy hormones and utilise your brain's own in-built drug platform but doesn't reinforce unhelpful and maladaptive movement patterns within your body. Some examples are walking and swimming.

Clinically based Pilates, particularly if run by a physio with an understanding of pelvic pain, can be a helpful and functional way to retrain these muscles and allow you to functionally exercise well. It can be the case sometimes that too much Pilates can be reinforcing lots of 'core' tension and other exercise forms may be more appropriate. This is something your physio can help to guide you through.

At the end of the day, if you are engaging in movement and exercise that feels good for your body, there is no need to stop, and if there are things you aren't sure about or know definitely contribute to flare-ups, it is worth exploring other options with your physio.

Extra resources

As Alison mentioned, your therapist should be able to tailor a treatment program to suit your constraints and this should consist of exercises you can do at home. There are a number of stretches designed to relax the muscles surrounding the pelvic area and you can find them on many websites like The Pelvic Pain Foundation of Australia. Try to do these daily—I personally incorporate these stretches into my morning routine and it feels like a nice way to start each day. Remember, it's not a quick fix but it does make for a good start in releasing muscle tension and cooling the central nervous system.

Start with some controlled, deep breathing. This will help relax the muscles and put your body in a state of calm. I call this going into butter mode. No, really. I do my deep breathing and I visualise my body going into a butter state, my muscles melting (relaxing). It works a treat!

Knee to chest

Start lying on your back with both legs straight and relax.
Bend one knee to your chest.
Hold an easy stretch for 30 seconds
  while breathing deeply into
  your belly.
Repeat the stretch with other leg.

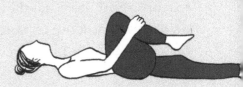

Knee to opposite shoulder

Start lying on your back with both legs straight.
Bring left knee to your chest and diagonally
  towards your opposite shoulder.
Hold an easy stretch for 30 seconds while
  breathing deeply into your belly.
Repeat the stretch with the right leg.

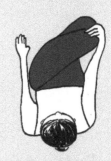

Foot and knee up

Start lying on your back with your feet on the floor
  and knees bent.
Bring your right foot to the front of your
  left knee.
Lift your left knee towards your chest.
Hold an easy stretch for 30 seconds while
  breathing deeply into your belly.
Repeat the stretch the opposite way with
  the left foot to right knee.

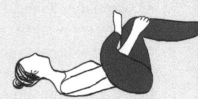

Knee over to hand

Start lying on your back with your feet on the
  floor and knees bent.
Left knee comes over your body to the floor near
  your right hand.
This can hold the knee down.
Hold an easy stretch for 30 seconds while
  breathing deeply into your belly.
Repeat the stretch the opposite way with the
  right knee to the floor on the left side of
  the body.

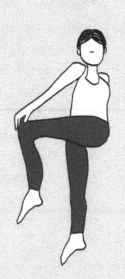

Child's pose

Start on your hands and knees.

Relax your bottom down towards your
  heels—your knees are wider apart; feet
  closer together. Your head can rest
  on the floor.

Hold an easy stretch for 30 seconds
  while breathing deeply into
  your belly.

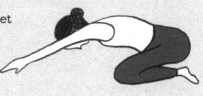

Flat frog

Start lying on your back with the soles of your feet
  together and knees falling apart.

Bring your feet comfortably close
  to your bottom.

Hold an easy stretch for 30 seconds
  while breathing deeply into
  your belly.

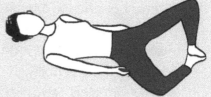

Happy baby

Start lying on your back with your feet
  on the floor and knees bent.

Grasp the inside of each foot—arms
  inside your knees. If you can't
  reach your feet, grasp the inside of
  each knee instead.

Allow your knees to widen apart.

Apply gentle pressure downwards.

Hold an easy stretch for 30 seconds
  while breathing deeply into
  your belly.

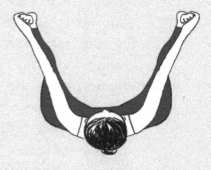

Adapted from the Pelvic Pain
Foundation of Australia

A mini pep talk on exercise . . .

I know, I know. When we're in pain, the last thing we want to do is exercise. Often our immediate perception or idea of exercise is something that is high intensity and triggering to our pain, so naturally we have a negative association. I'm not here to say, 'Let's go smash some sprints and burpees before a decathlon!' Personally, not my jam, but if you want to go do that, power to you. As Ali mentioned, there are a number of low-impact movements that work well for people with endo and they can do some pretty good things for us! Some benefits of exercise include:

- Increasing anti-inflammatory and antioxidant markers within the body.
- Reducing estrogen levels.
- Happy hormones! Honestly, I think this is the best thing about exercising. When I go on my walks, I do it to feel good, not to lose weight. Endo can be quite a hit to our mental wellbeing, but exercising is a nice way of producing natural endorphins and giving us a mood boost.
- Motion helps the motions! For real though, exercise reduces the time it takes for the food you eat to pass through your large intestine. In turn, this limits the amount of water that gets absorbed from your stool into your body. The less water that your body takes from your stool, the easier it is for you to pass it and the more regular your bowels become!

Top tips for movin' that bod

- Do something you enjoy! Maybe it's dance classes, aerobics, a swim or cycle. Abso-freakin-lutely stick with the exercise that makes you feel good because that's the first step to true health.
- Pace yourself. Especially if you are trying a new form of movement. It might take a bit of trial and error in figuring out the most suitable intensity and duration. Keep in mind this could also change throughout your cycle so keep track of what you're doing, when and how it feels.
- Don't compare yourself! Just because you see someone else with endo pumping some hard iron doesn't mean you need to. Everybody is running their own race.

What's the deal with yoga anyway?

Some of us endo warriors can't help but eyeroll when we hear this word because there's a lot of unsolicited opinions out there from people who do not have endo, but 'have a friend' whose endo was 'cured by yoga'. While this can never be true, I don't want to fully knock this practice because it does in fact offer some benefits. (Not a cure.)

In their book *Beating Endo*, Dr Iris Kerin Orbuch and Dr Amy Stein discuss the effect of yoga on the vagus nerve. The what? Don't worry, I had no idea the vagus existed either but turns out it's the longest cranial nerve in our body and look, she's a social butterfly! Vagus interacts with basically everyone and everything, linking the brain stem to the heart, lungs and gut. All the key organs know her and whatever we do, vagus has some sort of involvement.

Orbuch and Stein spoke with Dr Ginger Garner who said there are five mechanisms of pain that yoga can alleviate via the vagus nerve: inflammation, the sympathetic nervous system, oxidative stress, brain activity and opioid receptors. Dr Garner explains:

> The more we influence the vagus nerve through yoga, the less we experience inflammation. Where the constant perception of pain is concerned, yoga's influence on the vagus nerve can actually reverse the perception by combating the blood vessel constriction and muscle tension that chronic pain induces. All this plus its ability to influence the opioid receptors without pharmacological compounds make yoga's influence on vagus nerve activity incredibly valuable.

In 2017, Brazilian researchers randomly divided 40 women with endo into two groups: those practising hatha yoga and those going about their regular lives. For two months, the yoga group attended two 90-minute classes each week. At the end of the study when the two groups were compared, the women doing yoga reported significantly less daily pain, as well as an improved sense of wellbeing.

I'll leave this one with you but whether it be for movement or mindfulness, the concept of yoga is definitely a 'don't knock it until you try it' kind of thing when it comes to pain management and relief in pelvic health. If you do decide to try it, I'd suggest Hatha yoga as it is much gentler than the likes of Ashtanga. I strained a muscle during Vinyasa, lol. But, hey, each to their own!

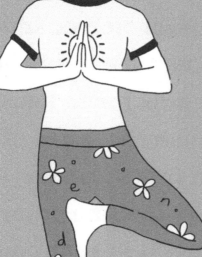

" One of the most difficult factors of this somehow isn't the gunshot-wound pain. It's the psychological pain that you experience. It's also the unknowing that really adds to the psychological damage. I think anytime someone is in chronic pain for so long, it's almost like there are phantoms living in there . . . even when you don't feel the pain, you remember it in your body and then you still kind of feel it. "

MAE WHITMAN

7

Mental health matters

So, you've been diagnosed with an incurable chronic condition after experiencing what has likely been years of pain and dismissal from medical professionals who have perhaps made you feel like it's all in your head, as well as a lack of understanding from those in your personal and/or professional life which in turn has made you feel like a complete burden, and now you're faced with the uncertainty and anxiety that comes with it all, like whether you can have children or if you will ever been pain-free. *exhales* It's a lot to take in, isn't it?

The pain of endometriosis doesn't start and end with your period. So often, we focus on the physical consequences of this disease, but it is important to also recognise the mental and emotional toll endo can take. Admittedly,

I never considered this until I attended the RANZCOG Annual Scientific Meeting in 2019. It's basically this big conference event full of workshops, discussions and keynote addresses concerning the OB-GYN world. There were a range of presentations including one session from Associate Professor Christina Bryant called 'The Role of the Psychologist in Chronic Pelvic Pain'. In Bryant's presentation, she explained the unique position that psychologists are in to address some of the key concerns of people with chronic pelvic pain and it was at this moment that I felt Extremely Seen. *Holy shit, endo has totally cooked my mental wellbeing.* Turns out that I'm not the only one feeling this way. A 2019 report conducted by the BBC in collaboration with Endometriosis UK found that out of the more than 13,000 participants, 94 per cent said that endometriosis had affected their mental health. Nearly 50 per cent stated they have experienced suicidal thoughts.

Sadly, I don't think anyone with endo would be shocked to hear these stats. Think about everything you've endured—that's going to *abso-freakin-lutely* affect your work, your relationships with others and, of course, the relationship you have with yourself. Endometriosis can bring about so many feelings and emotions, like the following.

Grief

- Difficulty accepting your diagnosis
- reduced quality of life due to the limitations that pain presents—losing opportunities
- mourning the person that you used to be and the relationships that may have diminished throughout the course of your condition

- unsuccessful attempts at conceiving
- cancellations and delays to treatments/surgery.

Anxiety

- Doctors not believing you and rejecting your symptoms/ pain
- infertility
- experiencing a new symptom
- the thought of being away from home and in pain
- uncertainty regarding the future, for example, having a job, a partner and/or family
- financial burden of the disease
- fear of pain arising at any given time
- fear of pain never improving
- fear of constant judgement (usually dealt with through concealment of disease)
- fear of conflict (usually dealt with through self-silencing).

Guilt

- Letting your colleagues down by taking time off or not being able to complete all tasks due to your pain
- letting your friends down by not being able to see them as often and missing special events due to your pain
- letting your family down by possibly having to borrow money for treatments or not meeting their expectations of success due to your pain
- letting your partner down due to lack of intimacy
- becoming dependant on others
- 'killing the mood' when you open up about your endo-metriosis struggles.

Confidence

- Declining self-esteem and belief that you can do anything
- negative relationship with your body due to changed appearance (bloating, surgical scars) and functionality (fitness, painful sex, etc)
- talking yourself out of pursuing goals or relationships
- externalised self-perception (self-judgement based on external standards).

Losing a sense of purpose

- Lack of independency and identity
- feeling that endometriosis defines you and the life you live.

Loneliness and isolation

- Not being able to go out with friends, family and/or partner
- feeling like no-one understands your pain or not knowing anyone else who has endo
- difficulty dating or making new friends
- internalising pain.

Medical trauma

- Being told by medical professionals that it's all in your head or that others have it worse than you, also known as medical gaslighting
- being misdiagnosed or declined the request to see a specialist

- bad reactions to drugs or examinations, especially without true informed consent
- repeated ineffective surgeries and complications
- unnecessarily removing reproductive organs
- being deemed hysteric or difficult by clinicians.

These are just *some* of the ways in which endometriosis can impact you mentally and the list is so huge that it really deserves its own book. And, of course, your mental state is going to influence your physical wellbeing. As Dr Pamela Stratton explains in the 2016 *Endo What?* documentary, there is a real pain cycle when it comes to endometriosis.

Pain causes suffering, suffering causes depression, depression can then feed back into pain and so, they are interacted on an emotional-physical level. But they're probably connected on a biochemical and mind-body level as well.

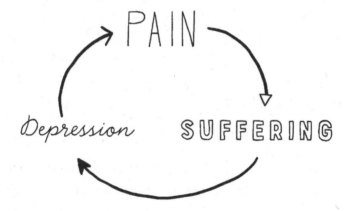

For all of these reasons, it is vital to include our mental health in the management of endometriosis.

But how do we do that? I'm going to take you through a few different ways, starting with the most obvious—a psychologist.

A psychologist has a role to play throughout your entire endo journey, from that moment of you questioning your pain, trying to find a diagnosis, accepting the diagnosis and the challenges that may come with it, for example, hysterectomy, fertility.

Psychologist versus pain psychologist . . . What's the difference?

Psychologists and pain psychologists are both allied health professionals who specialise in the treatment of mental health problems and human behaviour. But a pain psychologist focuses on the human behaviour *that accompanies chronic pain.* There's no right or wrong one to see, it really just comes down to the psychologist themselves and whether you feel they suit your situation.

Katie is 27 years old, from Melbourne and follows endogram. Unlike most people, it only took her a year to be diagnosed with endometriosis, but the process involved a great deal of research. One of the biggest discoveries she made was how beneficial a psychologist was as part of her multidisciplinary approach. She says:

It has honestly changed my life. My psychologist helped me deal with a lot of anxiety that came with having an endometriosis diagnosis, as well as the stresses before I was officially diagnosed. She gave me a number of strategies to help me deal with anxieties around the fear of what endo may cause me to miss out on—especially being in too much pain to attend social events and then let my friends or family down, or miss out on work opportunities, or negatively impact my studies. She also helped me realise that my pain was often worse when I was stressed, and the importance of making sure I do everything I can do to minimise general stresses in my life, and how that would help with my pain levels significantly, but in an indirect way. Things like making sure I exercise, eat well, drink a lot of water, get at least eight hours of sleep—all of the things that are important for your mental health that also happen to help endometriosis symptoms!

Katie has a unique perspective as she has also seen a pain psychologist, an experience she described to me as both amazing and confronting.

Through appointments with my pain psychologist, I had to deal with certain events and trauma in my past that turned out to be linked to the pain I was experiencing. The body has a way of storing and dealing with trauma that I had no idea about! Through some emotionally taxing but very rewarding sessions, I learned more about that and worked through a lot of feelings and can say I came out of it much more informed, sure of myself and comfortable with my past. This knowledge has also enabled me to help a few of my friends who have experienced similar situations and have talked to me about it, which I am grateful to now have the knowledge to do.

In addition to this, Katie's pain psychologist provided valuable insight on the links between the brain and the body, which is something that Katie first heard of in her regular psychologist appointments.

My pain psychologist taught me about the benefits of visualisation techniques in meditation, as well as giving me a lot of techniques to deal with the pain whilst it was happening. She taught me that the way you frame the pain in your mind matters. I recognised, with her help, that although I was experiencing pain, because we knew the cause of the pain (endometriosis, of course) and we knew that the pain wasn't putting me in any danger, it was not a threat, so it is better if I can deal with it in a more positive way. My favourite thing that she taught me to do was to literally talk to my uterus (out loud) when I am in lots of pain, and to say to it that 'I know you are feeling pain now, it's just endometriosis pain because the cells similar to your uterus lining are growing places that they shouldn't, it is okay and it's not a dangerous pain.' I used to feel really silly when I did this and it definitely makes my partner laugh, but I think it really helps!

Elise, 28 and from Melbourne, was diagnosed with endo in 2011 and we actually had our second surgeries on the same day by the same specialist! For Elise, she found a regular psychologist to be the perfect fit. Elise says:

I would recommend shopping around for psychologists if you don't feel you connect in the first few sessions. My psych isn't a chronic-pain specialist and that may be helpful for some, but she was just what I needed. She helped me stop feeling guilty about my illness. Being a high achiever, I had negative feelings around work and not being good enough or productive enough. I also had issues with bailing on social events and feeling like I couldn't keep up with my friends. My psychologist made me see how self-critical and downright bitchy I was being to myself and helped me find ways to turn my thinking around. She made me realise how important looking after myself is. She let me vent, justified my angst and introduced me to coping tools to assist with my anxiety—mainly based around understanding my thoughts, breathing and meditation. I saw her up until February 2020, before she went on maternity leave and now, I see a new psych who is also wonderful. Seeing a psych turned my life around and I think was one of the main tools I acquired that truly started the healing process for my endo.

While it is super encouraging to hear the experiences of Elise and Katie, it is an unfortunate reality for many people with endo that ongoing consultations with a psychologist or pain psychologist are not financially possible. With that in mind, I want to suggest some ways in which you can help manage your mental health on a budget.

Suss out government assistance

This will vary depending on where you live, but in Australia, if you have lived with chronic pain for at least six months you may be eligible for a rebate through Medicare for allied health services to help manage your condition. If you are experiencing mental health issues associated with chronic pain, you may be eligible for a GP Mental Health Treatment Plan. At the time of writing this book, Medicare rebates are available for up to ten individual and ten group allied mental health services per calendar year to patients with an assessed mental health issue who are referred by a GP. For more information, visit the Australian Government Department of Health website and speak with your GP.

Support groups and helplines

You will see this pop up a few times throughout the book because they are honestly going to help you *so* much. If you can afford to see a psychologist or pain psychologist, a great way to find local recommendations is through the experiences of others shared on support groups. If these kinds of consultations are outside your budget, utilise online support groups instead because they can also serve as a safe, interactive space for you to seek advice and connect with people going through the same thing. These support groups can feel like free therapy!

If talking to someone on the phone is more your thing, there are a range of 24/7 hotlines around the world that allow you to receive immediate support anonymously. Even some endo organisations like QENDO and Endometriosis UK have their own phoneline that you can call to speak with a trained volunteer who has personal experience with endometriosis. While they cannot provide medical advice, they can help answer any questions you may have concerning the condition and serve as a listening ear. You can find both their numbers in the Recommended Resources section of this book.

Journalling

When I say journalling, I'm not referring to those after-school 'Dear Diary' entries we would often write about our BFFLs and crushes then slam shut and padlock before anyone could see. BUT if you want to do that, I fully back you.

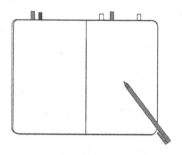

For real though, journalling is a therapeutic form of self-expression that can improve your mental wellbeing by helping you address problems, fears, and concerns. By tracking symptoms daily, you can come to recognise triggers and learn ways to control them better. Journalling also creates a safe space for identifying and resolving negative thoughts. Even when you don't feel positive about your situation, you can still be positive to yourself and journalling is a great way to practise that healthy kind of self-talk.

Mindfulness

Mindfulness is all about being engaged and aware of what is happening in the present moment. No distractions, no judgement, just self-observation and acknowledgment of the effects that certain thoughts have on your body and mind.

Let's say you're sitting in a park, for example. Instead of sitting there and thinking about your last doctor's appointment, what to cook for dinner and when you are due for your next period, you are thinking about ... sitting in the park! Feeling the grass beneath you, the sunshine radiating from above and taking in the sights and sounds. You are fully present, not thinking about anything else in your life, just what is happening right here, right now. By teaching the mind to be present, we are teaching ourselves to live a life that is more mindful and less reactive.

Mindfulness is poppin' right now. In 2019 alone, there were 1449 studies on mindfulness published in peer-reviewed scientific journals. It seems like a pretty basic concept on first glance, but mindfulness is not a habit that can be developed overnight. If you are seeing a psychologist, they may like to try Mindfulness integrated Cognitive Behavioural Therapy (MiCBT). It's pretty self-explanatory, MiCBT blends mindfulness with some basic elements of Cognitive Behavioural Therapy (CBT) in order to help improve the way we feel and change unhelpful behaviours. However, MiCBT focuses more on changing the process of thinking, not just the content of our thoughts. As outlined by the MiCBT Institute, this is done over four stages:

1. **Personal stage**—notice and let go of unhelpful thoughts and emotions in order to address life's challenges successfully. Develop insight and realise that you don't have to be prey to every thought that enters your mind and every emotion that you feel.
2. **Exposure stage**—apply these self-regulation skills in situations that you might be avoiding, which will result in an increase in self-confidence.
3. **Interpersonal stage**—develop better interpersonal understanding and communication skills when encountering tense situations with people and learn to not react to how someone else may respond.
4. **Empathic stage**—increase your capacity to be kind to yourself and compassionate with others in your daily actions, this leads to a greater sense of self-worth and deeper care for others.

Another way to practise mindfulness is through meditation. Find a comfortable position, focus on your breath and, if you need assistance, fear not: mindfulness is only a swipe away! There are dozens and dozens of phone apps out there that specialise in mindfulness meditation. It can be a bit overwhelming to navigate but here are a few to get you started:

- **Smiling Mind**—a free Australian meditation app that has been created by psychologists and educators and is designed for both adults and kids.
- **Headspace**—described as 'meditation made simple', this app has a very personalised approach in allowing you to pick sessions that best suit your mood and lifestyle. It requires a paid subscription but starts with a ten-day beginners' course.
- **Calm**—a very popular American app for sleep, meditation and relaxation. Like Headspace, it involves a paid subscription but for that you get Harry Styles narrating a sleep story so . . . *throws money*

While we have seen the topic of mental health become more normalised in recent years, there is still a stigma attached—especially when it comes to seeking help. Doing so is not a sign of weakness or that you are broken. I know many people who are generally quite positive and successful but still take time to speak with a psychologist or turn on a mindfulness app. Why? Because happiness doesn't end sadness. We are all works in progress and just because someone is high functioning, it doesn't mean they aren't struggling in some way. As my friend Claudia once said, the reality is that endometriosis is a scary, all-encompassing mind-fuck and we shouldn't feel ashamed to admit we aren't always coping.

" I don't know who needs to hear this but just because you have a chronic illness doesn't mean you're lucky that people date you. You're still that bitch. And they're lucky that you're choosing them too. **"**

LARA PARKER

8

Let's talk about sex, bby

Sex. It's supposed to be a steamy little word, isn't it? One of excitement, curiosity and pleasure. Fun and adventurous. The ultimate way for humans to connect. I wish those things were my initial thoughts but usually my mind is occupied with anxiety and dread. I get tense. I think of the need to be drunk in order to deal with that painful, pulling sensation. Or the building pressure from my vaginal canal that quickly extends to my bladder, sometimes even my abdomen. It can get so bad that even for hours afterwards, I'm curled up in foetal position, deflated and full of frustration.

- 'Being punched deep in your intestines.'
- 'An open wound being rubbed with salt.'
- 'As if my uterus is trying to climb up my body.'

- 'Pulling, like knives cutting in.'
- 'An abrasive dull pain, like if someone pushed on a serious bruise but worse.'

Those are some ways my endogram followers have described their painful sex. For many people with endo, this is our normal. No endless, hot and heavy action. Just uncomfortable attempts that we would rather get over and done with.

For the majority of my sexual life, I just thought I was the problem. That my body was failing me by not being cut out for sex and that I simply couldn't handle it. I had no idea endometriosis existed, let alone its strong association with painful sex. Up until my diagnosis and research I, like so many, accepted this as something I would just have to deal with.

As we learned earlier, the medical term for pain with penetrative sex is dyspareunia. When there is penetration during intercourse, the endometrial implants within the pelvic cavity can stretch, pull or push. And you bet ya bottom dollar it hurts. Our bodies then respond to this pain by clenching up which unfortunately promotes more pain. The sensitivity of the nerves is heightened and the next thing you know, the brakes slam and sexytime suddenly comes to a halt. Didn't take long, hey?

All of this can have such a devastating impact on our self-esteem, our body image and our relationships. You can't help but feel useless, unfulfilling to your partner and, frankly, like a sad sack of shit. But there is hope! Improving sexual function is a legitimate health issue and a complex one that requires attention from physical, psychological and social perspectives. Therefore, sex is a key component in the management of endometriosis and, thankfully, there are people out there who Just Get It! Like Chantelle Otten, a Melbourne-based psycho-sexologist, scientist and relationship expert. Thanks to her strong social media presence and approachable nature, Chantelle has helped normalise some of the conversations surrounding sex, particularly when it comes to pelvic pain. So here she is to answer some of your (literally) burning questions.

Why should people with endometriosis consider adding a sexologist to their multidisciplinary team?

Sex can be difficult to manage with endo due to pain, fatigue and discomfort, so a sexologist is here to help you manage those difficulties. One of the key indicators of endo is pain with sex, and that can be devastating for a lot of endo warriors and their partners. It's my job to help manage this with them, minimise discomfort and open their minds up to great ways they can have pain-free sex! It's really about redefining what sex means to you and how to create the best journey for you.

What can people expect from their first consultation with a sexologist and how does it differ from a psychologist?

In the first session, we will have a really healthy conversation where I take a detailed history of your overall health, mental health and sexual history, plus establish why you are coming in for a consultation now. We then make goals, such as 'I want to have pain-free sex', and we work towards those goals together. A sexologist differs from a psychologist in that there is a lot (A LOT) of collaboration and education about *sexuality*. Psychology is the study of the human mind whereas sexology is the study of sex and sexuality, but usually from a psychological background.

What are some ways in which a sexologist can help people with endo overcome the association of pain with sex?

As we have established, painful sex is a common side effect of endo, which is awful. But the great news is that there are numerous ways to alleviate the pain, and also to help manage intimacy expectations, so you can still have a fun, pleasurable sex life. Having an endometriosis diagnosis doesn't mean you need to lead a life of celibacy and my role is to provide support, education and empowering advice in overcoming this negative relationship between sex and pain.

Pain is a cycle, so if you have experienced painful sex, your brain associates that area of your body with feelings of distress and discomfort. The way in which we counteract this is through developing a pleasure cycle. I do this by working with a pelvic floor physiotherapist to see if we can adjust the tightness of your pelvic floor and also working with the mind around reconditioning that area so it is not associated with fear and pain.

What advice would you give to someone with endo who is single and having (or wants to have) casual sex?

Honestly, don't be scared to date and to have casual sex. I suggest you take the time to really get to know your body, what you like and don't like, so that you can lead your erotic encounters to make sure they are pleasurable, not painful. Then, just keep it real when you are on dates! Tell them that you may experience pain with penetration and the ways that you navigate around it. But *I beg you*, do not push through with having painful sex, because it will make your body tense up more and the pain will increase. If your sexual partner is not willing to accommodate your needs, then . . . maybe that is not the person for you. Considering it is casual sex, you have the ability to find someone who *will* make you feel like a babe and treat you with respect.

And for those with endo who are in relationships and struggling with sex?

It's okay for you both to feel a little disappointed if your sex life is struggling due to endo and your partner should be supportive and not pressure you. Sex is often the hardest thing to talk about with your partner so it's important to be kind to each other. Your pain, while absolutely valid, may lead to your partner feeling rejected and undesired. As a result, there may be some performance anxiety from both sides which can interfere with having fun in the bedroom. I believe you should see a sexologist (like me!) to help you navigate this, because it's a tricky topic for *anyone*.

Chantelle and Bridget's tips for an endo-friendly sex life

Communication is key

Communication really is the foundation of a healthy sex life. Experiment with your partner to find positions that don't hurt. From modified doggy-style and spooning to oral and anal sex. Even kink or roleplay! The way you share your fears and desires is important as well so be conscious of wording and if you get stuck, book a sexology session.

Penetration isn't the only pleasure

It's really about redefining what sex means to you and in many cases, penetration is just a no-go. This is completely fine; there are lots of people who have non-penetrative sex lives and still feel amazing and satisfied! Be open to changing your idea of sex and embracing other practices like 'outercourse', which is non-penetrative intercourse. This includes manual stimulation, pleasure products and oral sex. You can still orgasm from long, hot, drawn-out foreplay!

Let's be real, foreplay is the main play. Warming up is so necessary and it can start in many ways—whether that be a sensual massage with a happy ending or a huge make-out session. Remember that you are there to enjoy the journey, not just the destinations of penetration or orgasm.

Toys and tools

This is a particularly fun part! It's super important to explore other types of pleasure that are not intercourse focused and, luckily, the market is pretty huge when it comes to finding some great pleasure products, whether that be a clitoral vibrator, nipple clamps, anal beads or a male masturbator. Whatever tickles your fancy!

Another option is buying a product like Ohnut which controls the depth of penetration that a penis can have. Using a pillow or a sex wedge can also help control your positions and avoid angles that are typically painful. Beaded glass dildos can be cooled or heated—you may find a chilled toy can bring relief to an inflamed pelvis. It's as easy as popping one in the fridge or running warm water over it.

Finally, lube it up, bby! Lube makes everything better and the more the merrier. Try for a water- or silicone-based lubricant—water is super versatile while silicone is hypoallergenic, so most people won't experience a reaction.

Explore your erogenous zones

An erogenous zone is an area of the body with heightened sensitivity that can produce a sexual response when stimulated. The first area that springs to mind is, of course, our genitals, but there are so many throughout our body, such as your scalp, ears or even your inner wrist. Make a map of pleasure in your body, get to know these spots and tell your partner where to find them! It's the perfect way to enjoy more levels of intimacy.

- **Scalp**—Whether it's a gentle stroke or a playful pull, hair is the gateway to all those glorious nerve endings in the scalp. Don't forget that spot between the ears and neck for some soft caressing.

- **Ears**—A simple way to enhance some traditional mouth kissing is by lightly tracing the C-shaped outline of the ear with your fingertips at the same time. Or have a cheeky nibble of the earlobes, gently pulling with your teeth. Deep breathing into the ear is a winner if you love a bit of ASMR.

- **Nape of the neck**—All it takes is some running fingertips, soft kissing or breathing across the nape of the neck to make the whole body tiiiingle.

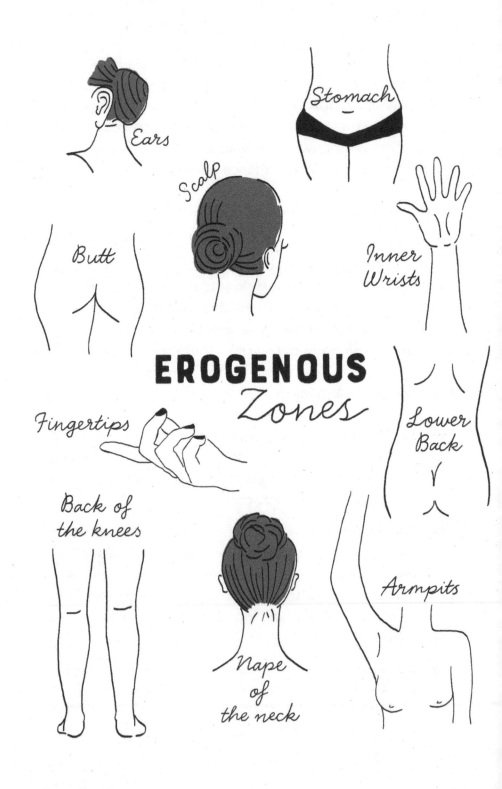

EROGENOUS
Zones

Ears

Stomach

Scalp

Butt

Inner Wrists

Fingertips

Lower Back

Back of the knees

Nape of the neck

Armpits

- **Armpits**—We know the armpits can be ticklish ... and sweaty. And hairy. But! They're still a sexy spot! Try rubbing an armpit in circular motions or do a little graze. Need a visual? Watch *Dirty Dancing*: Baby and Johnny have you covered.

- **Inner wrists**—Lightly caress them with your fingertips if you're feeling suggestive, or if you're already in the thick of it, a feather, kiss or lick can help take things up a notch.

- **Fingertips**—A gentle nibble or light suck is steamy AF, especially if eye contact is being held.

- **Stomach**—Given its close proximity to the pelvic region, the stomach is a total tease. Have fun with your tongue, fingertips or a feather to trace circles around the navel.

- **Lower back**—The nerves in the small of your back (sacrum) are connected to your pelvis, so this a particularly sensitive region for sexual stimulation. It's also a great spot to experiment with temperatures, whether that be with ice cubes or a heat pack.

- **Butt**—Often there is an immediate association with anal penetration, but less invasive sensations such as a light caress of the outside skin or even doing some gentle fingering can be a great way to activate those numerous sensitive nerve endings inside your anus.

- **Back of the knees**—An unexpected hotspot, the back of the knees is perfect for a light massage, tickle, kiss or lick. Even a gentle bite could set you off!

Timing

Did you know that the timing of your period can help identify what stage of your cycle is most painful? Some people may be friskier after their period whereas others are keen to get into it pre-period. It differs for everyone and may take some trial and error, but it is definitely worth tracking. To help with this, try a phone app like Flo or QENDO.

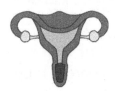

Hopefully these tips can help you navigate sex with endometriosis, but for a more personalised experience, booking in to see a sexologist like Chantelle is your best bet. And, hey, you don't need to be in a relationship or be having casual sex to see a sexologist, you can go purely for your own needs if solo sex is more your thing. Remember, the most important relationship of all is the one that you have with yourself. While it may feel like it at times, having endometriosis does NOT mean that you are broken in the bedroom. Sex is such an open concept and means different things to different people. There is sex that will suit you, it's just a matter of finding it. Having endo doesn't make you less loveable or desirable and it's a big Thank U, Next to anyone who dares to make you feel less than worthy. Whatever you do, do not settle. You deserve someone who loves ALL of you. That person will not be burdened by your pain, they will instead see it as strength. They are out there, I promise!

9

You are what you eat

If endometriosis was a food, I reckon it would be an onion.

I mean, it's not like endo has a strong smell, but there are plenty of eye-watering qualities about it. Not to mention the layers, it's never-ending! The more you unpeel this condition, the more you want to cry, and there's one particular layer that I have been dreading to touch until now—diet.

Gulps Yeah, that old chestnut. Turns out food is a big factor in how we manage our endo given the inflammatory nature of the condition. Therefore, what we eat can really influence our pain, whether that's fuelling symptoms or calming them down.

I'll be honest, dieting has never been my thing because I tend to associate it with restriction, pressure and misery. Growing up, I only saw the d-word used in reference to weight loss and being skinny. It was always about limiting or forbidding particular foods in order to meet society's expectation of what you should look like. However, as the years have passed, I have come to understand the true value of nutritional planning and ensuring our bodies are getting what they need for optimal health. When it comes to endometriosis, you are what you eat. If you're gonna smash down a highly processed, fatty feed, you're probably going to flare-up due to the inflammatory properties and formation of extra estrogen. Yet cruciferous green veggies (for example, broccoli, bok choy, etc) can help metabolise that excess estrogen.

Marika Day is a Sydney-based nutritionist and dietitian who specialises in gastrointestinal disorders and gut health. She's worked with many clients who struggle with digestive issues such as Irritable Bowel Syndrome (IBS) and those who are trying to overcome emotional eating, lose weight or manage symptoms of endometriosis and PCOS. Marika not only takes a bullshit-free approach to healthy eating but is a firm opponent of eliminating or forbidding foods from one's diet. And as a serial lover of chocolate, chippies and chicken nugs, that is music to my ears.

According to Marika, there are multiple benefits to incorporating a dietitian or nutritionist into our multidisciplinary team. Marika says:

> A dietitian can not only help you eat a healthier diet and help you make changes that are realistic and sustainable for you but they can help pinpoint any foods that may be acting as triggers for symptoms. A dietitian can also be a great source of credible knowledge on the role

of diet in endometriosis as it is easy to get lost in the misinformation found online.

Further to this, a dietitian or nutritionist can help determine your nutrition profile and eating behaviour. It's simply not realistic for me to provide you with a set of rules or commandments to follow because there is no one way to go about eating for endo. Everyone has different needs and varying symptoms but here's Marika to answer some of the most common diet-related questions that have been posed to endogram.

What can people expect from their first consult with a dietitian or nutritionist, and how do we know we are seeing the right person?

In a typical initial consultation with a dietitian or nutritionist, they will aim to get to know you and your circumstances in detail. This will often start with many questions about not only your diet but also your lifestyle, your medical history and any details about your day-to-day life, stressors and challenges that influence your food choices. You will likely be asked about your bowels and any gastrointestinal symptoms you experience. For me as a dietitian, it is about painting a picture of what the person is going through, what led them to this point and listening to them in order to pick up key details along the way. Within the first session, you and the dietitian will set goals and determine the order of priority if there are multiple concerns or goals. Often within the first session, the dietitian will also provide you with some information on how diet plays a role in the condition and will talk you through the plan for future appointments.

I believe, as with any medical or health professional, that the relationship you have with the individual is the most important thing. If you do not feel heard, if you don't feel comfortable sharing details of your life, diet or medical history with that person, then they likely won't be a good fit for you. The right person is the person who you trust, who has the knowledge to be able to assist you and that you feel supported and comfortable with. Also, it may be worth flagging with the dietitian before your appointment that you are coming to discuss diet and endo so they are aware and can let you know if they are not the best dietitian or nutritionist to speak to on that matter.

What foods should we avoid?

I am a strong believer that we don't need to completely eliminate foods or have forbidden foods, unless of course you are allergic. For many, this mentality can lead to bingeing on or overconsumption of these foods later, and in general a poorer relationship with food. It is still important, however, that we focus on choosing healthy foods that provide us with benefits most of the time. This means choosing more whole, minimally processed foods like fruits, vegetables, wholegrains, and lean proteins, and minimising the intake of refined and processed foods like crisps, sweets, baked goods, take-aways, fried foods, processed meats and sugar-sweetened foods or beverages.

Some people will find that certain foods or types of foods may increase symptoms of bloating, pain or lead to changes in bowel movements—these foods may include products high in lactose, like dairy products, or containing high amounts of wheat. It is important to note that this isn't the case for everyone and if you suspect that certain foods are causing a worsening of symptoms then working with an accredited practising dietitian can help you identify which foods may be causing this and the tolerable quantities for you.

What are the main foods that are considered endo-friendly?

While technically speaking, there is no 'endo diet' or 'endo-friendly foods', what we do know about endometriosis is that there is inflammation occurring locally and that consuming a healthy, anti-inflammatory diet, like the Mediterranean diet, may be beneficial. The Mediterranean diet is one that is rich in healthy fats like extra virgin olive oil, nuts and seeds and oily fish. It contains plenty of fresh fruits, vegetables, and wholegrains, while limiting red meat and processed or refined foods.

When it comes to digestive discomfort and symptoms of bloating or cramping, it is easy to quickly jump to blaming certain foods as the cause. However, with conditions like endometriosis, we want to ensure that foods aren't getting cut out unnecessarily. Endometriosis sufferers will often have symptoms of bloating and cramping as a result of the endo itself and the last thing we want to do is to burden someone more with a restrictive diet if it isn't going to offer benefits.

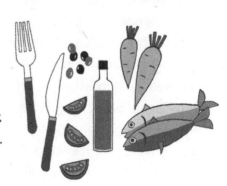

As for foods that might help relieve bloating or cramping, unfortunately there aren't any foods we can consume that will immediately relieve these symptoms however peppermint tea can be quite useful. When it comes to diet, it really is about eating healthy, balanced Mediterranean-style foods and minimising the intake of anything that may trigger symptoms.

The term 'low FODMAP' has been thrown around a lot in support groups. Could you please explain what that is and how it could potentially help people with endo?

The low FODMAP (Fermentable, Oligosaccharides, Disaccharides, Monosaccharides and Polyols) diet is a diet that eliminates foods that are high in short-chain fermentable carbohydrates. These types of fermentable carbohydrates, while incredibly good for our gut, can lead to excessive bloating, discomfort, pain or changes in the bowel for some people with Irritable Bowel Syndrome (IBS). It is a diet that is only intended to be followed for a short elimination period, followed by a reintroduction phase.

There is a large overlap in symptoms of IBS and endo and many people are diagnosed with both endometriosis and IBS at the same time or separately across their lives. It is for this reason that people believe that the low FODMAP diet is useful in endo and there is some research that is beginning to show that the diet is incredibly beneficial in the way of reducing symptoms in those who have both IBS and endo.

I think it is important to reiterate that it is not a diet that should be followed long-term, especially for those with endo, as it is a very limiting diet and restricts many healthy foods which are rich in prebiotics and provide health benefits. My suggestion is if you are thinking about going on this diet, speak with a dietitian who can help you move through the phases and identify which FODMAP foods are your personal trigger foods.

How can we keep an anti-inflammatory diet fun and interesting?

I think it really comes down to the perception of what an anti-inflammatory diet is. The best, most researched and healthiest anti-inflammatory diet on the planet is the Mediterranean diet and when we think of the Mediterranean diet it is incredibly diverse and abundant, especially with flavours, herbs and spices. An anti-inflammatory diet certainly doesn't need to be a boring diet, my suggestion is to look for some recipes in books or online to incorporate into your routine that are still delicious and fun while being good for you. It is a misconception that healthy food needs to be boring and flavourless.

There's not only an emphasis on what we eat, but also how we eat. What is the importance of gut/ digestive health, particularly with endo . . . and how can we achieve that?

If we think about HOW we eat, this comes down to optimising digestion. Often when we eat we are on the run, rushing a lunch break in between meetings or sitting in front of the TV at night, binge-watching our favourite show. Rarely do we take the time to sit at a dining table and eat slowly and mindfully.

This mindless eating can have a big effect on our digestion because when we are rushed or distracted, we often don't chew our food properly. Chewing is the first and a very crucial step in the digestive process. Without proper chewing, we are making the rest of our digestive system work harder to break down foods which can lead to bloating and discomfort. This is particularly true for stress as well: if your body is in a stressed state or sympathetic state, our digestion is affected. I highly recommend that everyone, not just those with endo, eat meals while sitting at a dining table with minimal distractions. Take the time to not just chew well but to *enjoy* the food.

How do we go about figuring out which nutritional strategies work best for us?

As with any nutritional strategy, there will always be a bit of trial and error to determine not only what suits your symptoms best, but also what fits in with your lifestyle and personal taste preferences or cultural needs. This is why I am a big advocate of working with a dietitian as it can often be overwhelming navigating the abundance of information online on your own and deciphering fact from fiction. Additionally, if some nutritional strategies are not carried out in a systematic manner or implemented properly, you may not see the full benefits and this is where I often find people jumping from one diet to the next, one strategy to the next, never getting to experience the benefit of any and feeling frustrated that nothing has helped.

How long does it typically take for people to notice a change within themselves?

When people make a change to their diet, we often see that within a week or two, they begin to feel better. Whether that be more energy, less severe symptoms or just feeling more confident within themselves. Ultimately, though, it will depend on the changes that you are making and your intentions behind them. If you make a change to your diet because you feel you 'should' and you hate every moment of that change, you will feel very different after a week compared with if you are excited to embrace new ways of eating, looking forward to trying new foods and recipes and are optimistic about the change.

Endometriosis is a costly condition to manage, do you have any tips for people who may not only be able to afford regular consults with a dietitian or nutritionist, alongside more expensive groceries?

Sadly, medical bills can add up and contribute pressure and stress to circumstances that are already stressful enough. For those who might not be able to afford consultations with a dietitian or nutritionist, it might be worthwhile looking to credible sources online for information or programs that come at a smaller cost. It is important not to end up spending money on misleading information or products which not only cost money but don't lead to positive outcomes either. I think the best approach is having a conversation with your specialist or GP about which avenues of care you wish to incorporate and prioritise and put the money to services that you not only value but have been shown in the research to provide some benefit.

What's the deal with . . .

Gluten

There is no need to eliminate gluten in endo, unless of course you personally find it is causing you digestive distress. Often when it comes to bloating and digestive symptoms, unless you have coeliac disease, wheat is the main culprit, not gluten. This means foods like spelt or rye are often better tolerated, even though they aren't gluten free.

Soy

Soy and soy products are rich in isoflavones which are phytoestrogens. Many people believe that, because of the role of estrogen in endometriosis, soy products need to be eliminated in order to reduce the occurrence of endo. When we look to the research, though, there isn't any evidence to suggest that cutting soy products provides either symptomatic benefits or reduces the likelihood of flare-ups. In fact there is some evidence that shows that regular consumption of soy products can actually reduce the risk of developing endometriosis.

Alcohol

In all circumstances, alcohol should be consumed in moderation and this is especially true for people with conditions like endometriosis simply because of the increase in symptoms like pain, bloating or cramps after regular consumption or consumption of large amounts. You certainly don't need to completely eliminate it but moderation is the key.

Coffee

There is no evidence to show that reducing or cutting coffee plays any role in endometriosis. Coffee does stimulate the bowels so can help people with bowel movements, which might be of benefit or cause troubles depending on how you find your bowels move normally.

Dairy

Like gluten, a common myth is that dairy needs to be eliminated for those with endo. For some people, the lactose found in some dairy products does increase digestive symptoms but for many this is not the case. Fermented dairy products like unsweetened yoghurts can actually offer many health benefits.

Sugar

It is a huge misconception that consuming sugar is bad for endo and that it must be completely eliminated. Yes, we should certainly limit our intake of refined sugars and focus on having a predominately whole-food diet, but there is no need to demonise sugar.

Supplements (for example, turmeric tablets)

Curcumin, which is the active compound found in turmeric, has been found to have anti-inflammatory properties which may be of some benefit in conditions associated with pain. This research hasn't been conducted in humans yet and so it is hard to definitively say whether taking curcumin is beneficial. We need some more data which informs us of how much is required, how long to take it for and, of course, if it does have a benefit in humans.

Intermittent fasting

Intermittent fasting can be carried out in many forms but when it comes to endo there is no benefit, unless of course it just simply is how you prefer to eat. Depending on the type of fasting you do, it can be completely safe but it certainly isn't a diet we recommend for everyone.

Again, it's important to reiterate that endometriosis is so individualised and everyone is going to have a different nutrition profile but hopefully these general tips can help get you started on some new strategies. Remember, it's about creating a plan that can hold up to the lingering nature of endo. There is no one, universal way to go about it. It will more than likely take time, a bit of trial and error and that is okay. Plus, food should be varied and fun! Just because we have a chronic illness, doesn't mean we can't still enjoy what we eat. So, if you don't mind me, I'm just going to finish my last nug . . .

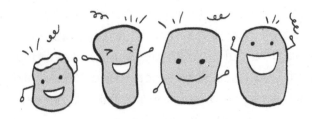

10

Complementary therapies

First, if you have made it this far, you definitely owe yourself a treat. Second, can you believe how much there is to do for effective management of endometriosis? I can hear my wallet weeping at the bottom of my tote bag, especially after mistaking the term complementary for complimentary. *What do you mean these therapies aren't free?!*

Despite this, remember that not everything works for everyone. Endo is an incredibly individualised disease. Perhaps you're already thriving in the bedroom or maybe food doesn't trigger pain for you. That's awesome! But if you're still struggling and wondering what else can be done, this chapter might help.

You may have heard of alternative therapies, but I personally refrain from that phrase when it comes to endo because

I don't think there is anything that should replace things like excision surgery or pelvic physio. We know that endo has whole-body effects, so it is important to incorporate a range of treatments that can work *alongside* each other.

As outlined by Dr Mike Armour for Endometriosis Australia, complementary therapy is an umbrella term that covers a whole range of therapies and remedies that are not part of mainstream medical care. It's an everchanging concept, as some therapies that may not have been previously embraced by GPs are now something that they would recommend for your health and wellbeing, for example, mindfulness meditation. Additionally, what is considered complementary can depend on where you live. For example, traditional Chinese medicine (TCM) is a mainstream practice in its homeland but deemed complementary in Australia where Western medicine takes the lead. However, more and more people are warming to the notion that Eastern and Western medicine can work in harmony.

I'm going to take you through some examples of complementary therapies and it's up to you whether or not you wish to pursue any for your endo. Endometriosis requires constant work and people respond differently to treatments. There is no one-size-fits-all approach to managing this condition and, as always, consult a healthcare professional. ☺

Chinese medicine

When I think of Chinese medicine, I think of my Nanna who had numerous joint issues and loved seeking relief by having teeny, tiny needles poked into her like she was a pin cushion. As a child, needles terrified me, so I was always scared to go with her to these appointments. I couldn't for the life of me understand why anyone would want to do this—how could you willingly take up to twenty needles AT ONE TIME? TO RELAX? It made zero sense to 8-year-old Bridget but it's a different story for 29-year-old me who now knows a thing or two about pain.

To help us navigate this ancient form of medicine is Lauren Gannon, a registered Chinese medicine practitioner and a member of the Australian Acupuncture and Chinese Medicine Association. After completing her Bachelor of Health Science (Chinese Medicine) degree at the Southern School of Natural Therapies in Victoria, Lauren undertook an internship in Taiwan at the Buddhist Tzu Chi Hospital. She now practises in Melbourne and has a keen interest in pain management, gynaecology, fertility and pregnancy as well as general health. I've been seeing Lauren for just over eighteen months and while it is different for everyone, I've personally felt improvements in my bloating and gut health as a result of acupuncture and Chinese powdered herbs.

As Lauren explained to me, Chinese medicine has an ancient history extending back more than 2000 years and incorporates acupuncture, herbal medicine, cupping and moxibustion as the main techniques.

Not all practitioners are trained in all modalities of Chinese medicine. It encompasses a holistic approach to health management. We cannot isolate one area of the body; we must analyse and understand the connectivity of the body to the mind and spirit.

Straight up, Chinese medicine has gone through some shit. My eyes widened as I learned from Lauren how this practice has overcome several battles throughout history, including the burning of the books and, later, the Chinese Cultural Revolution, where the practice was officially banned. 'Traditionally, a lot of the medical knowledge was passed down verbally, to reduce sharing of the information or "secrets",' she says. Today, it is taught as an extensive health science degree known as TCM.

The concept of TCM is based on a connection between mind, body and environment and aims to prevent and manage diseases. In regard to endometriosis, the therapy with the most supporting evidence is acupuncture, with one study finding that twice-weekly TCM acupuncture treatment significantly reduced pain after ten weeks.

Acupuncture involves the insertion of fine needles into specific points on the body. TCM theory explains acupuncture as a technique for balancing the flow of energy or life force, known as qi, believed to flow through channels in your body. By inserting needles into specific points along these channels, acupuncture practitioners believe that your energy flow will rebalance. 'We use acupuncture to encourage homeostasis, redirecting the body back to a state of balance and healing,' Lauren says.

Chinese medicine can explain the complexities of the human body in simple terminology. It stands back and looks at the wider picture. 'Blockages' can define, however are not limited to, any pain related condition. For example, a knotted muscle, sprained ankle, headache or menstrual cramps. If we look at the headache example, there will be blood vessel constriction at or near the site of discomfort. Hence why aspirin, a common *blood thinner, can be used for a headache. When you consume the aspirin, there is a chemical change and often pain relief. This is similar to acupuncture; we insert a needle, create a physiological change and the pain should reduce.*

This can tie in with numerous Western practitioners who view the acupuncture points as places to stimulate nerves, muscles and connective tissue. It is believed that this stimulation boosts your body's natural painkillers, known as endogenous opioids.

In Lauren's practice, an acupuncture session typically involves:

→ A detailed medical/health history would be taken, particularly in an initial consult. Discuss and identify the patient's main complaint(s) and what they aim to achieve from treatment. This can take between 30 and 60 minutes depending on complexity (fertility cases usually take longer). Treatment is focused on the main complaint(s) on a level of priority, working from top down.

→ A thorough menstrual history is very important. Establishing when the first period (menarche) started, when the pain started (if any), bleeding duration, the colour, texture/consistency, if there are any clots, and if there is anything that makes the symptoms better or worse. It's important to break things down and find out the details, like the time of the day in which symptoms are experienced. Even sleep quality, digestion/gut health and stress levels are all important factors. Looking for patterns helps determine the

Chinese medicine diagnosis and it requires a whole-body approach.

→ A return consult involves a much shorter check-in. It involves analysing the effectiveness of the last treatment and going through any current complaints/issues. Feedback is measured on a percentage level, for example, twenty per cent reduction in pain since the last treatment. Then the radial pulse is checked on both sides to help confirm diagnosis and abdominal palpation may also be performed. Another important inspection is that of the tongue. A tongue analysis helps to confirm diagnosis as well as analyse gut health and internal temperature. Important aspects of the tongue include the coat, size, marks, colour and texture. Pulse taking can also help determine which acupuncture points are to be used. Although speed is certainly an important aspect, it's not about measuring the heart rate. Instead it is about feeling the sensations of blood flow. Pulse qualities are often described as thin, wiry, slippery, soggy, weak, to name a few.

Then it's needle time!

A standard treatment with Lauren includes the insertion of approximately ten to twelve acupuncture needles. She explains:

Personally, I use needles 0.18–0.2 millimetres thin. Once inserted the patient lies on the table for 20–30 minutes to enjoy an 'acu-nap'. Acupuncture for endometriosis typically involves about four to six needles in the lower belly, a couple on the feet, two to four inside of the legs and inside of the arms and hands.

The acupuncture points are located at 'spaces in between things', meaning that we look and feel for a tiny gap to avoid vessels, nerves, tendons, etc. Often nothing is felt but sometimes a warming, slightly zinging sensation is experienced, which we call 'de q'. The acupuncture prescription (the selection of points used at the time of treatment) is determined by your Chinese medicine diagnosis and can depend on where a menstruating person is during their cycle, as there will be a different acupuncture points used during the menstruation phase compared to ovulation.

One of my personal favourite things about acupuncture is the heat lamp. Lauren uses it on the lower belly and the heat helps to increase blood circulation. It's such a warm, comforting sensation that puts me to sleep almost every time. I love lamp!

Another Chinese remedy to consider is herbal medicine. As Lauren explains, it requires a particularly personalised approach:

Chinese herbal medicine is prescribed based on a patient's Chinese medicine diagnosis. It is available via prescription only from a registered Chinese medicine practitioner as the herbs that we use are scheduled. Not all patients with endometriosis will be taking the same herbs due to the varying range of symptoms that may be present, however there is usually one shared pattern and that is blood stagnation. Blood stagnation refers to the idea that there is 'blood-like material', in this case endometrium-like tissue, growing in the 'wrong' part of the body.

Lauren advises that there is a set of parameters that must be met for particular herbs to be included or excluded in a formula:

This in itself makes each formula unique to the individual. Just like any medication that is prescribed, you should not share your TCM formula with anyone else, particularly as it will be made just for you. TCM formulas are often modified and there are strict guidelines as to what can and cannot be changed. This is because the herbs often work together to achieve a desired outcome.

There are various ways in which Chinese herbal medicine can be consumed and Lauren believes the more effective and convenient form is powdered.

Powder form is what we refer to as a herbal tea. It is prepared like an instant coffee to be consumed warm and the dose is typically twice a day. Herbal pills are also an option; however, it is not possible to modify these, therefore I would predict a slower response.

Lauren treats a number of patients with endometriosis and has seen improvements in pain and PMS symptoms such as headaches, fatigue and bloating. She has noticed changes to menstrual cycles, particularly when it comes to reducing heavy flows and clotting and, something that I personally noticed, improved gut health.

I see varying degrees of symptoms, from issues around ovulation, post ovulation and during the menstrual phase. Pain reduction is always a priority, as decreasing pain will increase quality of life and improve other areas such as sleep and mood.

So, how do we find the right TCM practitioner?

Find a practitioner that has a focus on gynaecological conditions. As a registered health modality, we cannot "specialise" in any particular area as such, however those that have an interest in/focus on gynaecology have undoubtedly completed additional courses to further their understanding.

Finally, cost can be a big factor in determining whether someone can access regular TCM sessions. Currently in Australia, Medicare does not cover acupuncture and only private health insurance rebates are available. Lauren's best advice if you cannot attend treatment is to incorporate the following lifestyle changes based on TCM theory.

Diet

Fresh food is the way to go! Eating organic where possible to reduce pesticide consumption and avoid processed food where you can. Also opt for more cooked, warm foods rather than raw and cold to support digestion—it takes your body more effort to break down cold foods so you may be more prone to bloating, passing wind or digestive sensitivity. Same goes for water, try to drink it filtered at room temperature. If you don't have a water filter, you can boil your water gently for five minutes and allow to it to cool. Otherwise, water-filter jugs are available at major supermarkets for about $30.

Ensure that you have optimum levels of iron and other essential nutrients that are vital in ensuring we feel at our best. Good ones to check include vitamin D, B12, iron, folate and zinc. You can get this tested from your GP as well as a hormonal panel, which is a blood test to check your levels for estrogen, progesterone, follicle stimulating hormone (FSH) and thyroid hormones. This test can help evaluate infertility concerns as well as possible abnormal bleeding and check for things like menopause and PCOS.

Lifestyle

Look around your home and consider removing pollutants like air fresheners, toilet spray and perfume. Most of these common household items purchased from a supermarket are hormone disruptors and/or act like estrogen (pseudo-estrogens). This can present harmful effects to your body and potentially trigger endometriosis pain. A research study from 1992 also confirmed a connection between environmental dioxin exposure and endometriosis. Opt for glassware containers over plastic and avoid scented or dyed toilet paper. You may also like to review other items like make-up, washing detergent, soaps, shampoo, etc. Switch to natural ones where possible.

Finally, when it comes to menstruating, try to slow down in life. You can do more vigorous exercise during the follicular phase and more gentle activities from the luteal phase until the end of your period.

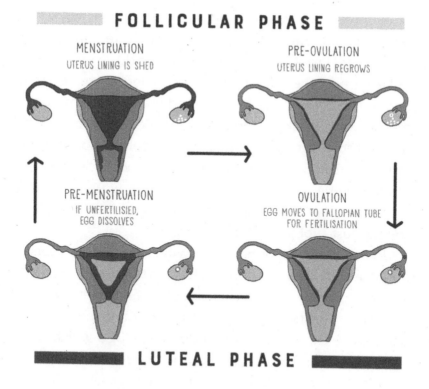

FOLLICULAR PHASE

MENSTRUATION
UTERUS LINING IS SHED

PRE-OVULATION
UTERUS LINING REGROWS

PRE-MENSTRUATION
IF UNFERTILISIED,
EGG DISSOLVES

OVULATION
EGG MOVES TO FALLOPIAN TUBE
FOR FERTILISATION

LUTEAL PHASE

Diagram of the menstrual cycle

Naturopathy

Admittedly, I've been scratching my head about naturopathy for a little while. I've always understood that it involves taking a natural, holistic approach to remedies and lifestyle advice, but I've never quite grasped what it is exactly that separates a naturopath from a dietitian or a TCM practitioner. All three professions have the same aim in improving your health but how do we know which one to see? I certainly couldn't afford ongoing consultations with *all* of them and it seems like some of their advice could overlap. The only way we can do a full comparison is by sussing out all three and to finish the puzzle, I needed to find a naturopath.

Like every other time I have been in doubt, I turned to my endogram community for help and many of them pointed me to Jade Walker. Jade is a qualified naturopath and herbal-tea maker with a degree in Health Science, and is based in Geelong. She also HAS endometriosis! 'I got my period when I was eleven years old and it wasn't long after that it became a monthly traumatic event. Pain was always the biggest problem,' she told me.

Jade had her first laparoscopy when she was 21 years old and was told she was 'all clear'. It wasn't until she completed her studies that she learned about excision surgeons with advanced training—and just how much can be missed. Jade underwent excision surgery in January 2020 which did, in fact, detect endometriosis, so if we count the diagnostic duration from her first period to this surgery, that is seventeen years. SEVENTEEN YEARS, Y'ALL. 'Going into my degree, I always hoped it would give me the answers to my debilitating pain. That's when I came to the conclusion that I likely had endometriosis with everything I was learning.'

Here's Jade to help us further understand the relationship between naturopathy and endometriosis.

What is naturopathy and what can it do for people with endometriosis?

Naturopathy is a holistic modality that utilises nutrition, herbal medicine, supplements and lifestyle habits to create individualised treatment plans. Naturopathy has evolved immensely over the years and is now a respected practice that requires the practitioner to complete a four-year Bachelor of Health Science degree to become accredited.

Based on these holistic principles, naturopathy supports people with endometriosis by looking at every area of the body and by not taking a one-size-fits-all approach. Where naturopathy really shines with endometriosis is helping to reduce pain and heavy bleeding by utilising specific evidence-based dietary measures and anti-inflammatory supplements and herbs. But as I see from working with many endometriosis sufferers, not every person's treatment aim is the same. For example, for one person it might be to deal with the pain, for another it might be fertility, and for another it might be to manage the constant bloating. Thus, naturopathy works with the patient so well, because we don't just give every endo sufferer the same cookie-cutter advice. With that said, we do have some key advice that every endo sufferer should follow to get the best results such as removing dairy and adopting an anti-inflammatory diet.

How does it differ from seeing a dietitian or a traditional Chinese medicine practitioner?

Put simply, a naturopath differs from a dietician by the addition of herbal medicine. But there are many types of dieticians and many types of naturopaths. So, the comparisons may vary. For example, some dieticians may be very meal-plan focused or disease-specific, adhering to Australian dietary guidelines and using evidence-based information.

While there are some similarities with TCM, such as herbal medicine, there are also differences in our approaches and philosophies. TCM has a particular focus on meridians and thermal natures of the body (to all my TCM friends, I'm sorry if I butchered that). TCM utilises herbal medicine, but also has a strong focus on acupuncture. Personally, as someone who has utilised TCM and acupuncture for my own endometriosis, I believe that naturopathy and TCM can be quite complementary to one another. A naturopath may have more of a focus on nutrition, use completely different herbs and really dig into every area of your life to find the missing links such as going over blood tests and doing further functional testing. Meanwhile, TCM practitioners utilise other techniques to assess the patient's body.

What does a session with a naturopath typically entail?

An initial appointment is typically one hour to go over your full health history. I get all new clients to fill out a lengthy intake form with as much detail as they remember from the day they were born to now, which helps us piece together the jigsaw puzzle that is their presenting condition. I also go over any recent blood tests, as the current standard reference ranges are not always best for optimal functioning, particularly iron, B12, thyroid and vitamin D. I can't tell you how many times I've seen people feeling flat and fatigued, and I take one look at their blood tests and they're depleted in almost everything. After assessing their history, diet, environmental factors and main health aims, I create a personalised treatment plan and prescription for them. I've also created an endo handbook for all my endometriosis patients that helps them understand their condition, along with all the key advice I've learned through research and my own experience. They will usually have their first 30-minute follow-up around three to four weeks later (particularly as I like to see how their period changes with the treatments).

Typically, treatment plans may run from three to six months depending on their individual goals and what else is going on.

Endo can be a costly condition to manage. Do you have any tips for those who may not be able to afford consistent appointments—anything they could do from home?

Absolutely. And this is something I can relate with a lot. Going through my own studies, being a broke uni student, I'd often get upset learning about all of these treatments that I just couldn't afford. This is why I love to 'overshare' on my Instagram with videos on what I do to help my own condition, so that people have a place to get started. Endeavour College of Natural Health has a student clinic, which is only $20 for an initial consult, where you can see a final-year naturopathy student. They are all under the guidance of seasoned naturopaths/lecturers, so you know you're in good hands.

There are also actions every endo person can take right now that could make a huge difference. I know it's hard, but eliminating dairy is important. Dairy contains the A1 protein which drives up inflammation. Just eliminating this one food group can be a game changer for many.

Ensure you have a healthy intake of omega-3 (particularly from oily fish sources like salmon, trout and sardines) which reduces inflammation. If you don't eat fish, supplementing is a good idea. The big five that often need to be removed are dairy, coffee, alcohol, wheat, and red meat. But full disclosure. I'm not perfect with avoiding these 100 per cent either (coffee, dairy and wheat are the main culprits I avoid). But the more you stick to it the better you will feel.

Ensuring you have good gut health can also make a big difference, as we now know that those with endometriosis have a higher presence of certain bacteria that drive up inflammation. So, ensuring you have regular daily bowel movements with plenty of dietary fibre and fermented foods like sauerkraut and kefir is great. You might also benefit from a temporary low FODMAP diet for two to three months, which may aid with bloating and IBS. Finally, herbal teas can also serve as a cost-effective healthy intervention, which is something I've created with much consideration of the common ailments I see clinically. Ginger, cinnamon and turmeric are the big three culinary spices I get everyone to incorporate to reduce inflammation and promote circulation.

How has naturopathy personally helped you manage your own endometriosis?

In every facet you can imagine! Reducing the pain has been the most challenging part and something I've had to work extremely hard on. But being able to manage my period without Naprogesic (period pain tablets) has been the biggest achievement. As well as that, I no longer have PMS or sore breasts before my period nor do I have several large clots. I have more energy. I know my body's cues when I haven't been sticking to the plan, and the rest of the time, I've got my digestion on track.

I used to always have severe 'endo belly' and could never figure it out. But I later realised I had Small Intestinal Bacterial Overgrowth (SIBO), which is linked to endo and for me was causing constipation. So, I treated that and my bloating subsided. Like all of us, I still have my bad days. I still fall off the wagon from time to time or go to town on a cheese platter. I still get pain, but it's more confined to one day and more manageable with herbal medicines and a TENS machine, rather than needing several days downing painkillers. The 'bad' experiences are much fewer and further between and I have the tools on hand to reduce those flare-ups to a manageable level.

So, there you go, you've now met a dietitian, a TCM practitioner and a naturopath. It's like one of those cocktail parties on *The Bachelor*. You've had some alone time with each and nobody was drunk or dramatic (sorry producers), but they did present some contrasting viewpoints so it's really up to you as to which advice you follow. Have a think before you hand out those roses. Maybe you'll pull a plot twist and go on second dates with all three? Power to you, my friend. I'm Osher, so I respect your choice either way. 😊

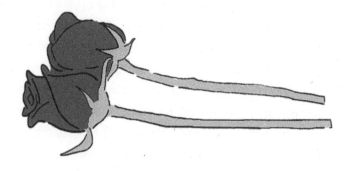

Cannabis

I personally had no idea about the use of weed to relieve endometriosis symptoms until I launched endogram in 2019. Before that, I just associated the plant with the film *Pineapple Express* and my very failed first attempt at using a shitty DIY bong in a friend's run-down caravan at the end of high school. I'm talking full juice bottle vibes with a cut-up garden hose as the stem—gnarly stuff. However, the more endo pals I have connected with, the more I have heard about the positive impact of cannabis in managing their chronic illness.

In the lead-up to my second surgery, I decided to seek out a few weed cookies. Choosing to have the IUD removed meant I would be returning to agonising periods and cannabis was something I had not yet tried to help combat that pain. I remember lying on the couch cautiously nibbling my cookie and being reacquainted with the taste that had me coughing my guts up fourteen years prior. The next 90 minutes was a waiting game, but it worked.

The pain became distant, as if my body just got up and walked away from it. I felt relaxed, warm and fuzzy. I also got the munchies, but I was able to retreat to my bed with a big smile on my face and, instead of waking up throughout the night, I had the most peaceful sleep. The only other time I have slept this well was after a binge-drinking session, but with the cookie, instead of waking up hungover, I felt refreshed.

After testing the weed cookies out for a few cycles, I knew it was something I wanted to stick with, so I applied for medicinal cannabis. I went through Tetra Health, a tele-health service provider, and within two weeks of applying, providing the required documentation and consulting with their nurse and doctor, I was approved. A part of me has felt a bit rebellious given the taboo surrounding medicinal cannabis, but I think it's an important conversation to be had, because I know I'm not alone in the way the plant has helped manage my pain.

What is it?

Medicinal cannabis, or medicinal marijuana are pharmaceutical products made from the cannabis plant, used to relieve symptoms of some medical conditions. People have different perceptions of the plant, mainly due to its use as an illegal recreational drug and the associated stigma. However, there's a pretty big difference between pharmaceutical products derived from cannabis for pain relief and the consumption of marijuana for the purposes of getting High As A Kite.

How does it work?

It all starts with the endocannabinoid system, otherwise known as ECS. This is a regulatory system comprised of various receptors, binding chemicals and enzymes. Its main function is to maintain balance and stability within our body (homeostasis, for my science peeps) and is important for a wide range of actions, such as metabolism, inflammation and immune function. The ECS is distributed throughout most organs in our body but is more prominent in the central nervous, immune and the reproductive systems of those who were assigned female at birth.

Medicinal cannabis can come in various forms, such as oil, capsules, patches, oral spray, gel/lotion, edible and in its raw state to smoke or vaporise. The active ingredients in medicinal cannabis are called 'cannabinoids' and the two main types that we see used in products are tetrahydrocannabinol (THC) and cannabidiol (CBD). THC is the one that gives you those psychoactive effects of being blaaazed but it is also used to treat symptoms such as pain, nausea and muscle spasticity. CBD is the same chemical formula as THC but the atoms are arranged differently and as a result, it *doesn't* get you high. CBD has potent anti-tumoral, antioxidant, anti-spasmodic, anti-psychotic, anti-convulsive and neuroprotective properties which are believed to help ease and alleviate signals of pain, anxiety and inflammation, so it stands to reason that it would have a soothing effect on the ECS for people with endometriosis.

Are there side effects?

Yes indeedy! Like all prescription medicines, medicinal cannabis products can have side effects. The extent of these side effects depends on the product type and, of course, it varies between individuals. Some symptoms may include:

- fatigue and/or sedation
- vertigo
- nausea and vomiting
- fever
- change in appetite
- dry mouth
- diarrhoea
- feelings of euphoria
- depression
- hallucinations or paranoid delusions
- psychosis or cognitive distortion.

What's it got to do with endo?

According to the Australian Government Therapeutic Goods Administration (TGA), most of the studies on chronic non-cancer pain involved using medicinal cannabis *in addition* to other pain medications and focused on chronic (long-term) rather than acute (short-term) pain. The studies specific to endometriosis are limited but the plant boasts a long history with menstrual-related pain, dating back to as early as ninth century Persian texts. It has been part of Chinese medicine since the fifteenth century. During Queen Victoria's reign in the nineteenth century, it was well known that the regent received monthly doses of cannabis indica for menstrual discomfort throughout her adult life and, although never officially confirmed, there is speculation that she suffered from endometriosis. Following 30 years of experimentation with the plant, the Queen's personal physician, Sir J Russell Reynolds, was convinced of its effectiveness. In 1890, Reynolds took to world-leading medical journal *The Lancet* to declare cannabis 'one of the most valuable medicines we possess'. He said the plant was 'of great service in cases of simple spasmodic dysmenorrhea', aka menstrual cramps.

While some stigma remains, cannabis is being more openly talked about and one of my closest endo friends, Georgia Stuart, has been particularly helpful in sharing her use of cannabis to treat her endometriosis, adenomyosis and anxiety. Based on previous experience, Georgia knew it could really help manage her symptoms.

The first time I tried cannabis for endo was in 2015 while I was travelling across America. I had some pain going on and found CBD gummies and edibles in a shop. I would take the gummies daily which helped my achy body so much! The edibles helped me sleep so well which is sometimes difficult with all the pain that I experience.

Now medicinal cannabis is a key part of Georgia's endo management. She says:

Cannabis has changed my life completely. I have been able to cut right back on pharmaceutical drugs which is a personal win for me. Ibuprofen gave me reflux, codeine made me so violently nauseous and Endone made me extremely itchy. I would often just choose to be in pain instead due to those side effects I experienced. CBD is incredible for my muscle pain and anxiety and THC oil helps my nausea, stomach pains and allows me to have a proper, deep, restorative sleep.

Georgia's positive experience echoes a few recent studies, including one published in the *American Health Affairs* journal that found 62.2 per cent of people who use marijuana do so for their chronic pain. In a 2017 survey conducted by the National Institute of Complementary Medicine (NICM) Health Research Institute, with the support of Endometriosis Australia and EndoActive, 484 female-identifying people with surgically diagnosed endometriosis were surveyed about the self-management strategies they used. Of the respondents, who were aged eighteen to forty-five, 76 per cent reported using self-management techniques in the past six months. This included the use of heat packs (70 per cent), dietary changes (44 per cent), exercise (42 per cent), yoga or pilates (35 per cent) and cannabis (13 per cent). Out of all of the self-management techniques, cannabis was rated as the most effective for managing pain. 'This kind of data provides us with a really useful jumping-off point because it looks like women are using it regardless of its legality,' Dr Mike Armour told triple j *Hack* in 2018. 'If people are using it anyway, we really should be looking at the effectiveness of this.' Despite this, Dr Armour advised against obtaining cannabis illegally, which leads to the million-dollar question . . .

How do I get it?

How you can obtain medicinal cannabis varies depending on where you live and the regulations of each country state/ county/province. It seems to be quite accessible in parts of America, and Whoopi Goldberg even has her own CBD range! In the UK, medicinal cannabis is legal but, disappointingly, the guidelines bluntly state that it should not be prescribed to those suffering from chronic pain. Here in Australia, the laws vary from state to state but doctors can legally prescribe medicinal cannabis through regulated pathways like the Special Access Scheme Category B and the Authorised Prescriber Scheme.

After Georgia's most recent surgery in 2019, surprisingly it was her gynaecologist who suggested that she look into obtaining cannabis legally.

> *He knew I experienced hellish side effects from pharmaceutical painkillers and referred me to a clinic. Unfortunately, they did not provide any Medicare rebates so after some research, I found a clinic on the Gold Coast with regular doctors that could prescribe medicinal cannabis.*

Georgia obtained the new referral and took basically a library's worth of supporting medical documents such as ultrasounds, ER discharge reports, surgery reports and photos, in addition to written correspondence from her doctor and gynaecologist about her condition.

> *The consulting doctor was actually shocked at all the supporting documents I brought with me. I thought it was going to be a lot harder than it actually was. She talked to me about my lifestyle, my conditions and how pain affected my life. She prescribed me CBD oil to take daily and THC oil to take when my pain was bad.*

Before Georgia could access these products, she had to be approved by the government and the turnaround was quicker than expected.

> *I was approved within one day and my prescription oils were sent to my local pharmacy. I have regular check-ups with my cannabis doctor about how I'm going with my prescriptions. Recently, she prescribed me flowers to vape when I'm waiting for the THC oil to kick in (which can take hours sometimes and results in me reaching for paracetamol) and this has helped so much.*

Georgia lives in Queensland where the laws for obtaining medical cannabis appear easier to navigate compared with other states. While she has been pleased with the process, there has been a financial disadvantage. Every month, Georgia could be spending anywhere between $280 and $550 on her cannabis and, for a university student, that's some decent coin. Despite this, she reckons everyone should have access.

I think there is a lot of room for improvement, but I do also feel that more GPs should be looking into the benefits of cannabis. CBD should be more widely available as it doesn't give you that 'high feeling' and it is extremely safe and effective in comparison with morphine, codeine, etc.

The cost of medicinal cannabis alongside other barriers is what makes so many endo sufferers turn to the black market. This means illegally accessing CBD or THC online, often through international websites. According to Professor Nicholas Lintzeris, an addiction medicine specialist at the University of Sydney, this is common. 'The legal system we've had available now has been in place for about four years, and in the early days, for the first couple of years, we had a very clunky system,' he told ABC Radio National. Professor Lintzeris was the lead researcher in a study on how Australians use medicinal cannabis for everything from chronic pain to mental health conditions. An online survey of more than 1300 people found that while cannabis is used widely for medicinal reasons, the vast majority of respondents don't get it from their doctor. 'It was very difficult for patients to be able to find doctors who were knowledgeable and interested, the products were quite expensive, the legal hoops were quite pronounced. There were lots of hurdles, paperwork and so forth,' Professor Lintzeris said.

What should I do?

While I am obviously pro-plant, I am not a medical professional and cannot determine whether medicinal cannabis is right for your situation. If you're not keen, then that's totally cool, but if you do want to find out more, you should go for it. For Georgia, research and education is key:

Make sure you look into state laws and call around to get quotes. If your doctor is against medicinal cannabis, find another one who will listen to your needs. I also found it really beneficial to document my experiences with pharmaceuticals and take these supporting documents to my appointments. Even research papers of the benefits of cannabis with chronic pain, there's no harm in being over-prepared. Don't stop trying because, as I have found, cannabis has the potential to drastically improve your life.

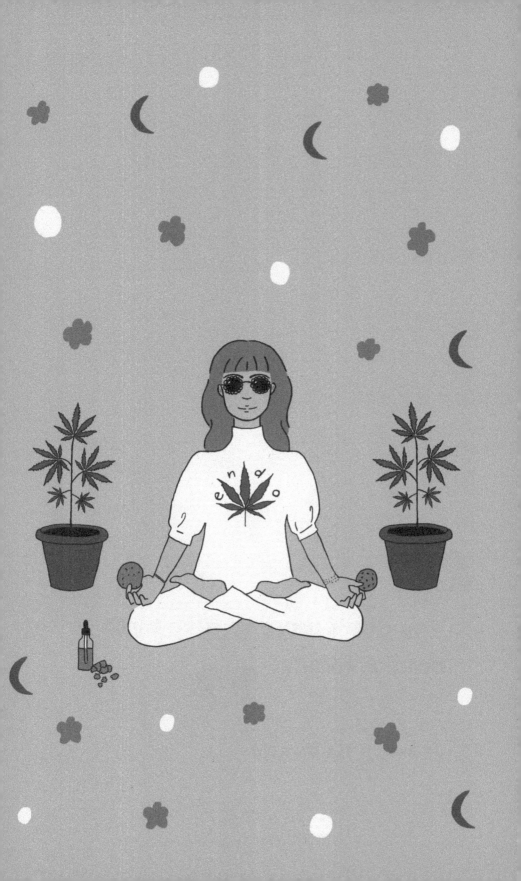

"

You don't have to give birth to have a family.

"

JESSICA MURNANE

11

Fertility and
parenting

Growing up, I planned to be a young mother. I remember one year at primary school athletics, our families were allowed to come along with picnic rugs in tow and cheer on as students eagerly competed in running races, long jump and shotput. I was about nine years old and my friend's grandmother was there, celebrating her 45th birthday. I couldn't believe she was a nanna, with her brightly coloured hair and fun jewellery. She was so hip for her age and had such an energetic presence that allowed her to well and truly keep up with everyone. She felt more like a cool aunty, if anything, the life of the party. I was so drawn to her and, in my head, I started to plan my future, as you do when you're in Year 4. It was then and there that I decided I would find a husband and have a child by no later than 24 because it sounded like a cool, young number and then when my children had children, I could be a cool, young grandma. It's that easy, right?

Wrong. A little thing called life happened. The years passed and I saw myself drift further and further away from the ideal of young motherhood. My aspirations evolved as I met new people and learned new things. I devoted much of my early twenties to a single life of travelling and blowing out a credit card to pay for it. I was emotionally and financially invested in experiences and making memories, not babies. My mid-twenties were a financially risky time as I worked my way up the music-presenting ladder, doing a lot of unpaid and casual work until I got where I wanted to be. I found myself in a serious relationship and then I was diagnosed with endometriosis. Now, I'm about to turn 30 and while I have many children in the form of plants, I very much lack tiny humans.

Isn't it weird how we give ourselves time frames to do things? I mean, I get having deadlines for tasks and projects (like writing this book!) but when it comes to traditional milestones, such as parenthood, the pressure to achieve by a certain age is *insane*. It's such a concerning societal issue that vagina owners face, as if our sole purpose in this world is to have a child. Especially for me growing up in a regional area, the general expectation was to find a dude, get married, buy a house and have a baby. Not that it's necessarily a bad thing, many of my friends have done it. But what if you don't want to? What if you *can't*?

For many people with endo, fertility is a tough conversation. Not everyone with endometriosis will struggle with fertility but according to Endometriosis Australia, up to 50 per cent will have difficulty getting pregnant. There are two main reasons behind why and how endo can affect fertility:

1. **Inflammation**—the inflammatory nature of endometriosis can impair the function of both eggs and sperm, as well as make an unsuitable environment for egg fertilisation, embryo development and implantation.
2. **Physical symptoms**—as the disease progresses, our anatomy can be distorted through scar tissue and adhesions, which can sometimes lead to blocked fallopian tubes and impact the passage of sperm and eggs through the pelvis.

Another way endo can affect fertility is pretty obvious: painful sex. If sex hurts, we're less likely to Get It On.

So, what actually constitutes infertility? According to the World Health Organization and the International Committee for Monitoring Assisted Reproductive Technology (WHO-ICMART): 'Infertility is a disease of the reproductive system defined by the failure to achieve a clinical pregnancy after twelve months or more of regular unprotected sexual intercourse'. For many people with endo, the struggle to conceive is hard to manage. Each period is a painful reminder that you are living with this chronic, incurable condition that is threatening the one thing you've probably thought about for as long as you can remember. It's also a reminder of the physical pain coming up, so that's fun. Then there is the sheer irony of doctors and friends telling you to get pregnant as a fix for endo when that's literally half the problem—you are trying, but you can't.

Sidenote: bringing a baby into this world is *not* a medical treatment for endo and it's pretty shocking to hear some professionals suggest otherwise. Sure, it may alleviate a bit of pain for some people, but it's not guaranteed. I had this conversation with Zara McDonald and Michelle Andrews on their popular *Shameless* podcast in 2019. You're either told to have a baby or have a hysterectomy, neither of which is an effective or proven way to heal endo, and they both sit at complete opposite ends of the spectrum. Where's the middle ground?

Fortunately, I'm looking good on the fertility front. Following my second excision surgery, my specialist was confident in my ability to conceive but, honestly, I'm still terrified. What if my endo grows back when I want to fall pregnant? Will it be painful? What if I have a miscarriage or high-risk pregnancy? My endometriosis has often made me feel so limited by my body. The pain has been unpredictable and, at times, out of control. How would I deal with that if I have a crying baby to attend to? My fatigue can really fuck me up some days as well—how could I possibly manage that alongside sleep deprivation? There's a lot of anxiety about the unknown.

Zara has detailed a similar sense of confusion in her and Michelle's debut book, *The Space Between*. A year after her endo diagnosis, Zara asked her gynaecologist about babies, to which she was told they would cross that bridge when they come to it.

> I found it peculiar that my future—my health—was now being projected in clichés that made little sense. How would I cross that bridge when I came to it when I didn't even know when I would be able to do the crossing? What if, by the time I got there, I had missed my window and there was no bridge to cross? Why couldn't anyone just give me a tangible answer to sit with now, so I didn't fixate on nonsensical metaphors about bridges and moats and fertility?

So, endo and fertility are bloody confusing. But let's try to make sense of it all together, yeah? The next question you may have is what can *help* fertility? For starters, excision surgery—physically cutting out the inflammatory endo cells—is a good start. Acupuncture is worth a shot too. A 2019 study found that acupuncture can boost chances of fertility by reducing stress as well as increasing blood flow to the reproductive organs and balancing the endocrine system. Third, we learned about pelvic physio earlier and if that can decrease the likelihood of painful sex then ... people are more likely to have sex! Woo!

If you are still struggling, it may be worth chatting to your GP who can provide a referral for fertility treatment like IVF.

In-vitro fertilisation, better known as IVF, involves injections to increase hormone levels and a surgical procedure a few weeks later to take eggs from the ovaries. These eggs can then be fertilised with sperm in a laboratory environment to grow an embryo. The embryo is placed in the uterus a few days later to help the conception process. The success of this depends on a few factors like age and how many eggs are retrieved and, while I have broken down the process in a very simple way, IVF is no walk in the park. It can be an overwhelming experience that can take both physical and emotional tolls, as well as sting your pocket.

Another option is egg freezing which is considered a kind of insurance for your fertility, helping out your future self. Egg freezing is similar to an IVF cycle, minus the sperm fertilising. To prepare for this treatment, a series of hormone injections are required before the eggs are retrieved. The eggs are then stored and when the patient is ready to go, their eggs are warmed and then fertilised with sperm. Sounds like preparing a meal, right? The Meal of Life! Except it's a bit more emotional than your average meal prep session, and you could have a few Michelin-starred meals for the same price.

Such an intricate process usually entails an out-of-pocket fee and potential 'storage' costs per year, but if you're not planning to pop some babies out anytime soon and want a form of backup when things look uncertain—and you're in a financial position to do so—this could be worth sussing out with your GP.

Finally, there is third-party assistance! We're talking egg donation, sperm donation surrogates, that kind of thing. There's a range of options and there's a range of fertility clinics too, so don't be afraid to shop around. This is something you have a huge investment in—both emotionally and financially, so it's important that you find a medical professional who is really going to have your back and be there throughout the process.

Alternatively, seeing a Chinese medicine practitioner or naturopath may help to prepare your body for conception.

Parenting

As you can probably understand, it's a bit hard for me to talk about this topic as I'm not yet a mother! Fear not, I have called on the wisdom of a familiar face within the endo community, Jessica Taylor. Jess is the president of QENDO. Despite initially forming in 1988 as a support system for people with endo in Queensland, QENDO has expanded into a powerful, worldwide community and a lot of that is thanks to the approachable, inclusive leadership style of Jessica.

The following pages may be triggering for some readers, particularly if you are having trouble trying to conceive. No words will ever do justice to those challenges and feelings of despair but if there's one conversation that needs to start changing, it's the narrative that a family is determined by our ability to give birth. It's frankly very dated and quite discriminatory towards not only infertile people, but also people in same-sex relationships and those who simply do not want to pop out a kid. There are various ways of forming a family and they don't have to be determined by medical procedures. Like endo, parenthood and family are not one size fits all—you are worthy and valid with whatever path you take.

Life as an Endo Mum, Jessica Taylor (President, QENDO)

Endometriosis was my firstborn. While friends of mine saw two lines on their pregnancy test, I saw flooding in my pad. While they charted the development of a new life, counting weeks then months, watching as it grew, I tracked symptoms, a seemingly endless array of them that never improved no matter how many doctors I saw. As they welcomed their child into the world, I welcomed a diagnosis, both filled with relief and then anxiety—how would I cope with this firstborn of mine?

As other people's babies grew into toddlers, my endometriosis needed constant monitoring. I watched it move through stages of development like a child going from purees to learning how to use a spoon, except I was the one with the mood swings of a three year old. I couldn't allow my condition to wander off, to roam unwatched;

it needed constant management and guidance, otherwise it was certain to become troublesome. I felt like a helicopter parent, a micromanager of my endometriosis, needing to know exactly where it was or what it was doing at all times.

But here's where our journeys take different paths. While others found watching their babies growing into children a precious time, I could not celebrate when my endometriosis marked a new milestone. Every new inch my endometriosis took over signalled another strategy I needed to develop, another treatment option to add to my ever-expanding toolbox. And whenever I looked at my swollen 'endo belly', so much like the belly of a mum-to-be, it was a reminder.

Endometriosis was my firstborn, but I was not yet a mother.

So, when I found myself pregnant, and then the mother of a beautiful baby girl, it isn't surprising that it was a unique journey, and yet oddly familiar. Being a mother with endometriosis is much like motherhood in general, a blessing and a challenge, a joy and a bit of a disaster all at once.

So, when are you going to have a baby?

The word 'mum' means something totally different to each and every person—and add some weight to this word if you're attempting to navigate your way through the fertility labyrinth.

The 'when are you going to have a baby' question is one that so many of us have fielded from family, friends and complete strangers in Woolworths while we're just trying to figure out which laundry detergent will leave our towels fluffy and bright without dooming the planet or our budgets. It's one of the most intensely personal questions that anyone can ask and yet it's often a topic of casual conversation.

When you have endometriosis, this question can sting just a little more than usual.

Perhaps you've been trying, unsuccessfully. Perhaps you've had miscarriages. Perhaps you're waiting because your pain is so unmanageable that your body just cannot cope with pregnancy, let alone motherhood. Perhaps you're in fact pregnant, but it's early and you're worried that it won't be viable. These are all the thoughts that occur behind closed doors, that people couldn't possibly know when they ask you this question and that's exactly why they shouldn't—no matter how kind or well-meaning they are.

Pregnancy

One of the only things many people know about endo when they are first given their diagnosis is that it could affect their fertility. On top of everything—the pain, the bleeding, the fatigue, the gut problems, the impact on your whole life—suddenly you're faced with the prospect that having children won't be easy, or even a given. That's confronting to hear, whether you're eighteen or thirty. Add another layer of complexity if you've also been diagnosed with adenomyosis or PCOS, or both for those who have the complete trifecta.

For some, becoming pregnant isn't difficult, for others there is some strategic planning and a few consults, maybe a fertility medication or two, and then there are others for whom achieving a viable pregnancy takes an army. Whatever path you take, finding out you're pregnant can be bittersweet when you have endometriosis. You live in a body that doesn't always do what it's 'supposed' to do and frequently does things that you wish it didn't. Your reproductive system in particular has proven itself problematic at best, untrustworthy and traitorous in other cases, and now you're supposed to trust it to carry a pregnancy?

One of the biggest myths associated with endometriosis is the notion that pregnancy will cure it or somehow improve it because it's nine months without a period—which assumes endometriosis is simply a disease of the reproductive system and not a whole-body illness. Those who have been pregnant with endo have mixed reviews on the subject, but for some the idea that pregnancy cures endo is the most laughable thing they've ever heard.

The early days of pregnancy can be overwhelming, some experience cramping that they fear is a miscarriage. The fear can be paralysing. The thoughts can race through your head at Olympic-swimmer speed. How many flutters have I felt today? Is she 'okay' in there? I remember calling the midwife (for the third time that week) concerned I couldn't feel any movement. The reassuring voice on the end of the line suggested that I drink orange juice or lemonade and count the movements. If it was what I normally felt or in line with her suggestions, we were okay. If you are ever concerned about your foetus, call your healthcare team. They are there to support you and help you navigate the (sometimes ridiculous) questions.

As a mum, my greatest fear is that my daughter may find out she too has endometriosis later in her life. I remember finding out the sex of our baby and sinking slightly inside, thinking, *A girl! But endometriosis can be genetic.* I dreaded the thought of my child going through what we do. This fear paralysed me and added anxiety to the journey. You may also be worried about how you will cope with a newborn. It is okay and normal to feel all of the feelings. Consider writing down daily affirmations to help you respond to your feelings.

The act of writing or journalling can help to actualise your thoughts.

Pregnancy is a totally different experience for each and every person—and for each pregnancy too! There are millions of books you can read, but here are a few key tips that helped me as a soon-to-be-mum with endometriosis:

- People with endometriosis often feel stretching, cramping or even shooting pain.
- It is okay if you don't trust your body but try to be kind to it and grateful each day for how far you have come.
- Make plans and organise as much as you can so that you are prepared for life with a baby and how you might manage your disease and a baby. Who in your support network can help?
- Develop a birth preference document instead of a birth plan. This can avoid further frustration with your body if your plan doesn't play out how you imagined it would. A birth preference document encourages you to consider your preferences around pregnancy and birth and prepares you for multiple scenarios should you need them.
- You can still flare and bloat, even during pregnancy. This can be tricky if you are not able to use your tools the way you used to. Keep moving. Motion is lotion and gentle movements will help your body stretch and adjust as it needs to. A warm shower, massage and moving through active birthing positions can help your body even more.
- It's normal to distrust the ultrasound. For people with endometriosis, we haven't had the greatest experience with scans, and I was really nervous the scans on my

unborn child missed or didn't pick up on key defects or issues. Talk with your sonographer or doctor about your fears and have them show you the images of the little bladder filling and emptying, the four chambers of the heart working together. Count the fingers and toes three times if you need to. Do what you can to understand your baby and focus on the facts.

Birth

The waves, the contractions, the surges. My body knew how to handle this deep and raw pain after years of experience. I am not saying that endometriosis and labour pain are the same, because every birth is unique and everyone is different, but I will say this: I knew how to handle the pain. Throughout my active labour, I breathed and moved my body, just like I do when working through an endometriosis flare-up: with heat, showers and moving my pelvis. I feel like endometriosis prepared me mentally to work through the process of labour and into becoming a mother.

The birthing experience is different for everyone. Most importantly, this is a time for you. Endometriosis has taught you that you know your body better than anyone else. You are your own advocate. Talk about your fears. Endometriosis has prepared you to understand your body.

The baby manual

You would have heard time and time again, 'Babies don't come with a manual'—maybe not, but they do communicate their needs to you. Endometriosis taught me to listen to and understand my body and I encourage you to do the same with your baby. They may not talk yet, but they do understand you on some level. They understand your energy, they understand your touch, they have been with you for nine months. They know you. It is up to you to understand and learn who they are.

Some parents don't always feel close to their baby right away and it's common to take time to feel comfortable in this new role. I remember the first time I was alone with my baby, just fifteen minutes after she arrived Earth-side. I sat there looking at her, thinking, *Wow, you are now a person I need to get to know*. I learned to understand her different cries and what they meant. I allowed her to be who she was, and I continue to respond to and follow her cues even to this day. Having something in your life like endometriosis, where you have very little control over your good and bad days, puts you in a unique situation. You can apply this patience, knowledge and experience to motherhood.

Endo Mum and managing your endometriosis

So, here you are. A new mum with engorged breasts, tired eyes and a baby who should be sleeping but isn't. Those early days are a total blur now that I look back and reflect. It was coming to terms with the fact my body achieved this and for the first time in my life, I was grateful for my body. I was grateful to my uterus!

When looking after someone else, it is important that your needs are met first. There is a reason why flight attendants instruct you to put on your own oxygen mask before anyone else's. A similar principle can apply to motherhood.

Here are some tips to self-monitor:

- know yourself—you know your own mind and body, listen to what it tells you
- allow yourself to recognise when it is too much—don't be hard on yourself
- contact a person you trust and feel comfortable to share your feelings with
- don't be afraid to admit when it's too much or it's not a good time for you
- write down a few things that help you lessen stress and anxiety levels.

When it comes to managing motherhood and endometriosis, two key areas come to mind: physical wellbeing and emotional wellbeing. It is here that you really do need to become an expert in developing your toolkit of resources and information to manage the mental load.

Physical wellbeing

Your physical wellbeing is essential to recover and replenish your body after conception, pregnancy and birth—and I don't mean working out three times a week. It is very common for mothers to be postnatally depleted throughout motherhood, regardless if you became a mother one, five or ten years ago.

It is time to invest and rebuild your physical wellness as much as possible. Postnatal depletion is not a new term, but one that is not widely known or spoken about often. It's when you are severely deficient in fundamental minerals and nutrients that are lost after birthing or carrying a child. Some people never replenish the fundamental nutrients and minerals needed to function and manage a condition like endometriosis throughout motherhood. Without the replenishment of essential nutrients, your body will struggle to manage inflammation and your condition.

If you read one other book this year, please look into *The Postnatal Depletion Cure* by Dr Oscar Serrallach. This book is a practical guide to replenishing your body after producing a child and will have positive impacts on managing your endometriosis too. It has been my best friend since becoming a mother and I encourage everyone in my life to read it.

Have you ever heard the phrase, 'Sleep when the child is sleeping' and laughed, thinking, *Yeah, right, I have so much to do around the house; I need to schedule appointments, cook dinner, plan work . . .* I wish I had understood how important this activity was in my early months of being a new mum. Sleep in those early days is even more beneficial for someone with endometriosis. Sleep helps to clear toxins, repair damaged cells, recalibrate your senses, produce restorative hormones such as dehydroepiandrosterone (DHEA) which boosts immunity, cognitive function and so many other good things your body needs. In addition, sleep throughout the early stages of motherhood is particularly important for someone with endometriosis because this is when your body does most of its detoxification and the gut works on absorbing and breaking down the foods you have eaten.

Emotional wellbeing and mental health

To some degree, anxiety or worry is normal when you are pregnant or a parent. Some will experience postnatal depression—please know, this is more common than you think. Recognise, accept and talk to someone early. You need mental strength to manage your baby and endometriosis.

You might be managing hormonal therapy or new treatments for your fatigue or pain while managing motherhood. It is really important that you seek support and be kind to yourself, more than you have ever been before. As a mother with a toddler, I found giving her small tasks such as combing my hair, finding my heat pack or sitting and reading a book is helpful. It might be an option for you to be open and honest with your children about how you are feeling. They might surprise you with how understanding and forgiving they are. I remember feeling really guilty not being able to play with my daughter due to a flare-up. I explained to her that I had a stomach ache and sore lower back. She promptly offered me a teddy bear to cuddle and sat next to me with a book, and told me, 'It is okay, I am here to help you.'

You might worry you will miss a netball match, dance recital or soccer game because you are in bed with a flare-up. It can be really overwhelming being a mum, so it's important that you check in with yourself and be kind to your body. Asking yourself the following questions throughout the day will help you manage your emotional, mental and physical health:

- Have I had enough water today?
- Am I straining or clenching my pelvis?
- Have I taken four deep breaths in and out today?
- Do I need a five-minute timeout to myself?

Remember, you are doing the very best that you can.

12

Work and study

Work

I'm just gonna put it out there, working with endometriosis sucks, from the guilt of calling in sick, the discomfort of trying to explain why, the anxiety of reducing hours and therefore losing income to wondering how you are going to make rent for the month or even afford groceries for the week. The fear of judgement from your boss and colleagues as you have no choice but to hand your work to someone else, again. The agony of pushing through a flare-up because you either cannot afford a day without pay or you don't want to let your team down. And then someone says, 'But you don't look sick . . .'

I'm quite privileged in my current role on radio. Sure, hosting a live, national show requires a certain energy, so sometimes it is really hard to show up and switch on when my pelvic palace feels like she's on fire. But the beauty of radio is that no-one *sees* you. I don't need to worry about wearing a restricting, ill-fitting uniform. Instead, I can rock up to the studio in whatever feels comfortable and, yes, that absolutely means trackies! I can be hunched over the microphone with a heat pack tucked into my pants and you'd never know. It's certainly not easy, but I know it could be worse. I've experienced worse. Like that time that I mentioned earlier when I was working my retail shift, crippled over the counter waiting for my regional manager to come and take over. Or in my previous role as a travel agent, squirming in my desk chair with a heat pack tucked under my uniform as I typed relentlessly to lock in airfares before my deadlines. I even had one lady return to my store to gift me an electronic heating pad after a Sunday morning consultation in which I gave terrible service because I was experiencing such excruciating period pain.

Plus, if there was anything good to come out of the pandemic, it would be the fact that I can do all my show preparation from home (read: on the couch with blankets) and hit the studio when it's time to go on air. I'm lucky to have flexibility and understanding from my employer on the days that I have to call in sick. They get it, but it wasn't always the case.

Anything but splendid

One month before my diagnosis in 2018, I was in Byron Bay for our Splendour in the Grass broadcast. Splendour is arguably Australia's biggest festival, it's our equivalent of Glastonbury or Coachella and for years triple j has broadcast from the festival site. We set up a radio station in a tent backstage to share all the action with those at home who couldn't snap up a ticket. While it's super fun having an all-access pass and chatting to some big names, it's not all glamourous.

In what I can only describe as So Bloody Typical, I got my period just as Splendour was starting. My uterus has always had this really good tendency to schedule shark week at the most inconvenient times, as if it were watching me and thinking, *Well, well, well. Looks like Bridget is ending her seven-day working week with a huge schedule at Splendour, let's spice up that stress with some cramps and clots!*

I was rostered to present the evening slot of the festival broadcast, so my start time was around 1 p.m. One of the days I was also pencilled in to do a field cross at 12.45 p.m., which, on first glance, doesn't seem like a huge deal because it is only fifteen minutes before my start time. However, the problem with this was the carpooling situation. Our accommodation was about 40 minutes from the festival site and there were only two times the cars went to site, 9:30 a.m. and 1 p.m. In order for me to do this 60-second field cross, I had no choice but to be onsite at 9:30 a.m. Instead of being able to use my morning off to rest with my heat pack and prepare my crampy body for the twelve-hour day ahead, I had to be onsite three hours early with no access to a microwave and just a plastic chair to sit on. For anyone who deals with bad period pain, you can imagine how those three hours would feel like a lifetime.

I messaged the team chat twice in the lead-up to see if there was any way I could swap my field cross with another presenter, only to be told that the cross would stand. Like many times throughout my diagnosis journey, I tried to suck it up, but it didn't take long for people to notice how much I was struggling. My then boss, who seemingly missed the group chat, asked me why I didn't swap with someone. Our technical producer spoke up in my defence: 'She DID ask to do that, twice.' I made it through the gruelling fifteen-and-a-half hour working day but that one incident has made me extremely anxious about returning to or working at festivals. It really affected me and I dread the thought of being in that situation again. I also can't help but wonder if the outcome would have been any different if I already had received my endo diagnosis—medically backed confirmation that my pain was the result of a legitimate condition. To everyone at the time, it just looked a bad period.

Nearly two years later when I shared my struggle returning to work from my second surgery on Instagram, I received this comment from a girl called Kasey:

> *I introduced myself to you a few years ago at Splendour and you were so lovely to me and then later I found out through your Instagram that you had the most horrendous pain that night. No-one would have been the wiser though because you were so kind and cool.*

It was a pretty bittersweet thing to read. On one hand, it was a nice reminder that, yeah, I'm strong as hell and can mask my pain like a pro. On the other, it was sad to remember that I was given no other choice. Sharing this experience with you is by no means an attempt to drag my employer, but I want you to know that this kind of shit can happen anywhere, to anyone. It doesn't matter what job you have or how well-known you are, working with endo is inevitably a challenge and there are going to be times where you're working alongside people who simply don't get it.

Performance anxiety

Take a look at American actress Mae Whitman, for example. In a recent interview with *Glamour* magazine, Mae revealed her struggle with being in pain on set and the fact that it wasn't taken seriously by the people she worked with. 'It's very hard. It's almost like you forget that you do have to then go be on camera. I felt like so much of my experience was about trying to manage and push down my own pain, push down on my own experience and be like, "I'll deal with this later."'

Mae had experienced symptoms for years before receiving her endo diagnosis and despite the validation it gave her, it has still made work prospects difficult to manage. She said:

I literally can't schedule things in advance. Like, it's almost a joke. And even now—I've had surgery and I'm much better—I still can't do it. Because the symptoms that I still have from endometriosis pop up out of nowhere. And even though it's not the horrible pain anymore, it's insane bloating, nausea, extreme fatigue, super-nervous panic attacks. And it makes it impossible because my cycle is all over the place. It's never regular. It's so frustrating because it makes you appear unreliable. People think you're just flaky. People think you're impossible to get a hold of, that you're not good at your job, you're not professional. I've had to sort of learn how to set up boundaries, which are probably good to have in one's career anyway.

Someone else who knows this feeling all too well is Jacinta Parsons, who broadcasts downstairs from me as an afternoon host on ABC Melbourne. For a few years now, I have dubbed Jacinta as my 'radio mum' because prior to hosting her own show, Jacinta worked for triple j's sister station, Double J, as well as being music director for Local Radio. For many of us, Jacinta became this nurturing figure who we could all turn to. In fact, she was one of the very few people I could confide in when I was told I had to move to Sydney in 2018 but had to keep it secret for two months. Little did I know, Jacinta was also battling an invisible illness, Crohn's disease.

In her article 'Pandemic has highlighted just how fragile we always were', published in the *Sydney Morning Herald*, Jacinta details her own battles with chronic illness in the workplace and the struggle for it to be taken seriously.

> If you come to work with a flu, or with a back that you've put out, the structure of the workplace supports you to resolve this issue and come back when it's all better. But there are no structures that meaningfully support an illness that is ongoing.

Jacinta lost nearly a decade of her career to her illness and had no choice but to work through her pain.

> What I learned to do, very skilfully, was hide my symptoms. I learned how to use my voice, to make the stream of air that travelled out of me so consistent, that nobody could hear the wavering pain beneath it.

Although she achieved her lifelong dream of becoming a radio presenter, she writes that she has 'no faith that our systems are built to cater for the chronically ill, and that vulnerability frightens me'.

Leave it alone

Another spanner in the works is sick leave. In June 2019, research by EndoActive and Ernst and Young found that endometriosis costs the Australian economy a whopping $7.4 billion a year in lost productivity. That's a conservative estimate, by the way, according to EndoActive co-founder Syl Freedman, who told triple j's *Hack* that this research only took into account time off work and underperformance due to illness. The report also found that 60 per cent of endo sufferers use their sick leave to manage their endometriosis, which doesn't at all surprise me. Endometriosis forces you to look at your leave balance from a completely different perspective. If I wake up feeling snotty or with an upset tummy, I need to consider if it is something that I can actually force myself to push through, because the endo pain always takes reign. Even when COVID-19 made its way to Australia, I was in full freak-out mode. I knew I didn't have the sick leave to cover me should I catch the virus, as that balance was reserved for my second surgery. I'm constantly thinking ahead, while it's rarely a thought that crosses the minds of my non-chronically ill colleagues. Imagine not having to worry about this kind of thing? I could never!

So, how does one work with endo? It all sounds so hard, and it is! But it is possible. I mean, in a perfect world we would all have incredibly supportive and flexible workplaces that would accommodate our illness but, more often than not, we have to put the effort in making our jobs more manageable. Everybody's situation varies—there are so many different kinds of jobs and we all have limits in how many hours we can do. For this reason, I can't give you super-personalised advice, but hopefully these general tips can help improve your working environment.

The Conversation

Having The Conversation with your boss and colleagues about your endo can be really hard and it's completely your choice as to whether or not you feel comfortable to disclose this information with them. I know many people who are open about it and I also know others who don't bother because they don't believe it's worth doing. However, while employers have a duty of care to their employees, it is the employee's responsibility to communicate with their boss. The level of detail you share about your condition is up to you (they probs don't need to see your operation photos) and your employer cannot share this with anyone else without your consent as it is private information. There are some employment contracts that mention the need to inform your employer if you cannot uphold your job requirements—in these instances, it would be really beneficial for them to know why that is the case.

If possible, make the conversation face to face so you can get a sense of their reaction and adjust the direction of the conversation if necessary. It could be worth doing some role-playing or planning out some different ways the talk could go, so you feel prepared to tackle it from numerous perspectives. Having a face-to-face chat also allows you to answer any immediate questions they may have.

Approach the conversation in an open manner and try to frame it as positively and optimistically as you can. This might sound weird, but from my experience talking to my bosses, I have found that wording can really influence their response. If I need to talk to them about a problem, I always try to offer solutions. For example, when I approached work about moving back to Melbourne, instead of saying, 'Hey, I hate Sydney, so I want to move back to Melbourne next year. Can we make that happen?', I tried something more like, 'Hey, I have really appreciated this experience in Sydney and have learned so much, but I feel that returning to Melbourne would improve my performance drastically. I've thought about the ways I feel this could benefit both myself and the station, and some suggestions as to how we could make this work. I'd love to explore these options with you and I'm happy to answer any questions you have.'

Can you see the difference? You want your boss to recognise that it's something you have really thought about from all angles because you, my friend, are a diligent legend! So, when bringing up your endometriosis, you want to go about it in a way that could be like:

> I wanted to talk to you because I think it's important that you are aware of a condition that I have called endometriosis. It's a chronic, whole-body illness where tissue similar to the lining of my uterus grows in other places and it affects me in a few ways [include some symptoms]. Here is some information that will hopefully help you gain a better understanding of what endo entails. I have thought about some processes we can follow to ensure that I can continue to work to the best of my ability [include some suggestions]. I would really love to hear what you think of these options and I'm happy to answer any questions. I'm looking forward to

making this work and as always, I value your support and feedback.

I would highly recommend downloading an information sheet from Safe Work Australia called 'Supporting workers with endometriosis in the workplace'. This sheet was prepared in accordance with the National Action Plan for Endometriosis and it helps employers understand the disease and identify reasonable steps they can make to help workers manage their symptoms. Endometriosis UK has set up a similar model called the Endometriosis Friendly Employer scheme, which enables employers to work towards improving support and developing work environments where all staff are comfortable talking about possible practical adjustments that could be of benefit.

You could also print a brochure or flyer from your local organisation—these are usually available as a PDF from their website—or even pass on articles about public figures who have endo. If you think it would help, you could ask your specialist or GP to write a letter to your employer that explains your endo and how it may affect your ability to work.

In terms of making suggestions, this really depends on your work and the extent of your endo. One thing I would consider is whether or not you can do part of your job from home. COVID-19 has forced many people to adjust their routines and adapt to working from home and, while it has been stressful for many, it has been music to the ears of many chronic-illness sufferers. If you have had to work from home recently, it could be worth opening that conversation with your boss as to whether it is something you can continue doing beyond the pandemic, or just on those days where you are in pain. According to the Fair Work Ombudsman, flexible work in Australia is available to employees upon request after they have worked continuously for an employer for a twelve-month period.

If you are unable to have this conversation with your employer in person, email is fine, but it could be beneficial to hit up some online support groups for advice on how to go about this. Alternatively, if your employer has one, call its Employee Assistance Program (EAP) for further guidance.

Know your rights

Legislation is different in every country so the best thing to do is print your contract and get to know it and how it relates to employment law! There will be important info in there regarding termination, sick leave and other work requirements so, if conflict arises, you can refer back to that for clarification. If you believe your endometriosis has led to discrimination, harassment or bullying within the workplace, the first thing to do is refer to company policy which should outline a process you can follow for complaints. If there is a HR representative available, contact them for clarity as some of these policies can be hard to dissect, but if you feel that you cannot speak with them confidentially or it will not be taken seriously, hit up an external party, for example, Fair Work Australia. Try to get responses in writing as it is much easier to refer back to and, as always, there are online support groups where you can seek advice and learn from the experiences of others who have gone through a similar thing.

The Vermilion Project

Tori Hobbs had been working in the healthcare industry for over four years before they were diagnosed with endometriosis and adenomyosis. One year prior, Tori was forced to take a lot of sick days due to their symptoms and, as a result, they encountered microaggressions, exclusion and animosity from their managers and co-workers. 'I was forced to leave my job due to the negativity, bullying and isolation I was experiencing, but I've since learned about my entitlements as a disabled worker and I've been able to find working arrangements that suit me.'

Although they were able to find new work, Tori often reflected on the experiences with their previous employer and wondered why they didn't know about the workplace laws that were in place to protect them.

> I grew frustrated at the circumstances I found myself in. Why was I not supported by my managers? Why was I told to go to Centrelink when I cried in front of them about the fear of not being able to provide for myself and my partner? How is it that I was made to feel alone, unproductive and worthless in an environment built on providing care to those who are unwell?

Growing up as an Indian Tamil migrant in Australia, Swathi Sundaram has had her fair share of discrimination based on the colour of her skin. 'I have been spat on and harassed but I would still regard having to justify reasonable adjustments to manage painful periods as one of the most demoralising experiences of my life.'

While completing her law degree and working in law firms, Swathi suffered from bouts of debilitating period pain and was severely overworked by a system that did not view her invisible illness as worthy of consideration. Despite feeling broken by her experiences of battling ableist workplace policies, Swathi was determined to ensure this did not keep happening.

Based on their lived experiences with juggling invisible illnesses and earning a living wage, Tori and Swathi decided to take matters into their own hands. They fused their love for law, healthcare and advocacy by launching The Vermilion Project, a collective aiming to create better personal and professional lives for people with chronic illnesses.

We believe everyone should be able to earn a living wage whilst feeling safe, supported and empowered in their workplace. We want workers with chronic illness to be knowledgeable about the laws that protect them, and we want them to know that they're entitled to the support we didn't have.

Alongside researching and gathering information from workers with chronic illness to better understand their needs, The Vermilion Project also independently reviews policies and procedures at an industry level to identify gaps in protecting workers, aiming to advocate for change at a systemic level. And this is only the start!

We're working on a series of intersectional self-advocacy workshops targeted at career-seekers and workers to ensure they have sound legal knowledge, self-advocacy, allyship and effective management strategies for when issues may arise in the workplace. Our goal is to protect, inform and empower workers so they may not only participate, but flourish in their social, professional and health journeys.

To Tori and Swathi, it's pretty clear that change is long overdue and that empowering people with chronic illness to manage their workplace issues benefits everyone—employers and employees alike.

Capitalism is built on the labour of people, but when you can no longer contribute in a way that is seen as 'fruitful' or in a way that is advantageous to your employer, your value appears to decline. However, your level of productivity does not have a bearing on your right to survive. Everyone has the right to earn an income, to access adequate healthcare and to not only survive, but thrive.

Be prepared

Create a checklist of things you need to have at work in times of a flare-up. You could include:

- pain medication
- heat pack—if you can, try to purchase one with a Velcro strap so you can wear it while moving around!
- stick-on heat pads—to avoid burns, wear some high-waisted underwear with them
- your 'urgent medical notice of endo flare' card—more on this on p 213
- if they work for you, a slim TENS machine that can sit discreetly under your clothes. Or if you're comfortable showing it off, werk that TENS, baby
- water, because hydration is #1 and you need something to help wash those painkillers down, duh!

Listen to your body

I know you probably just want to push through the pain, especially if it's threatening your pay cheque but if it's at the point where you can hardly function, you need to put yourself first. It's not worth creating extra stress on your body and the pain will probably continue to worsen. Take that time to rest or eventually your body will force you to.

And, listen to me!

You are doing the best you can. I know you are. Don't let your productivity define your worth and always put your health needs first.

Study

When I look back on my life, I always consider 2011 my favourite year because it was my first proper taste of freedom. I moved to Melbourne for the first time to study a Diploma of Visual Merchandising which, by the way, I have done a big fat amount of nothing with. I eagerly signed myself up for student accommodation that overlooked Glenferrie station. I broke up with my first boyfriend and was strangely excited to downgrade from my luxurious queen-size bed at my parents' home to a king single because it made me feel like I was well and truly a university student. Same goes for the lack of oven in the kitchen because, let's be real, are you even a student if your diet isn't goon, tinned tuna and instant noodles?

The university lifestyle is a thrilling notion but, in reality, it isn't the most endo-friendly life, given it usually involves a poor diet, excessive drinking and pressure to have a thriving sex life. Not to mention the workload, trying to stay focused and motivated when you're fatigued or feeling like your organs are rolling in barbed wire. It's not ideal.

However, there are a few things that may make studying with endo a bit easier. Massive shout-out to my endogram community for helping me put these together, many of whom are going through this stage of life right now!

Tell your tertiary/further education provider you have endo!

This is so important because they are in a much better position to help you than you may realise. Here are some ways in which they can help you:

→ **Access/Disability plans and Special Consideration**—don't feel ashamed to look into these plans, they are there to help and if you qualify, you could be granted extensions for your assignments. Just make sure your lecturers, professors and tutors are across it. They may also allow you to spread out your classes as opposed to doing several on one day, which may really burn you out.

→ **Student services and counselling**—most universities have student associations and their sole purpose is to support YOU! Utilise them!

→ **Health services**—consult your on-campus health service and advise them of your endo because they can be your extra backup if you ever need it.

→ **Online lectures and tutorials**—these are so common now anyway because of COVID-19 but speak with your teachers about the possibility of making this more accessible should you need. Come examination time, they may even allow you such things as bringing a hot water bottle or taking rest breaks. Have a chat with them, they are there to help you succeed.

If you are looking at going to university but are concerned about the amount of contact hours on campus, it could be worth exploring the possibility of part-time study as opposed to a full-time study load. Plus, some universities offer online correspondence courses that you may find more manageable.

Diarise your pain and plan ahead

So many of my followers suggested this one. Keep a diary so you can track where in your cycle you experience the most pain as you will likely detect a pattern. Use this pattern to help schedule your study around the good days. If possible, smash out as much work as you can when you are feeling good, so when you do come crashing down, you can allow yourself time to rest. Keep in mind, if it gets really bad, you should always put your health before study.

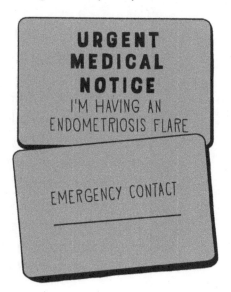

Be prepared

The same checklist for work can be used for uni. Pack medication, a strap-on heat pack or stick-on head pads, a TENS machine (if they work for you) and it could also be an idea to purchase an 'endometriosis emergency card'. Jump onto Etsy and search those three words and you should come across this yellow card you can purchase for a few dollars and it's basically a card you can pull out of your wallet and show people if you suddenly flare-up and need assistance. It's perfect for those times you're in a larger setting with lots of people, such as a lecture theatre.

A quick word for my high school pals . . .

This is without a doubt the most crucial time to be learning about menstrual wellbeing, pelvic pain and conditions like endometriosis. Being equipped with information and having the potential to fast-track a diagnosis can be life-changing for young people dealing with this pain.

If that's you, I want you to listen up, cos Big Sister Bridge over here has got some advice:

→ **Don't be ashamed**—period pain, heavy periods, whatever it is going on downstairs for you, is nothing to feel embarrassed about. It's real, it's important (just like you!) and it's not your fault.

→ **Communicate**—this can feel super daunting but it's so important that you chat to your parent/s/guardian about what you are going through so they can help you. Who knows, they may have gone through the same thing or know someone else who did! If they're not across endometriosis, send them some links from your national organisation. They may also be able to help obtain a letter from your GP to give to your teachers should you require any time off, homework extensions, etc.

→ **The same goes for your friends**—I know it can feel weird or like a taboo topic, but we need to normalise these conversations because endometriosis is too common to be kept quiet. Plus, your friends could also be experiencing the same thing and feel scared to bring it up. You could be opening a vital dialogue that can lead to a wonderful support system. If you are worried about them feeling grossed out, show them endogram. You are the exact reason why I made this account!

→ **Be prepared**—like you would at work or uni, put together a little endo/period kit to store in your schoolbag or locker so you are prepared at all times. You may have to seek permission to have painkillers at school but other things like pads, tampons and stick-on heat pads don't need approval and they're really handy.

I would also encourage you to speak with your health coordinator or school nurse about the possibility of an education program visiting your school to talk about these topics. Here are a few options:

Australia

In 2018, the Pelvic Pain Foundation of Australia launched the PPEP Schools Program. I literally squealed when I read the announcement because if this kind of program had existed when I was in high school, I swear my diagnosis would not have taken twelve years. PPEP stands for Pelvic Pain, Endometriosis and Periods and it's an interactive and informative one-hour session that allows students to learn more about these three topics and talk about any concerns they have regarding their own pain. As of June 2020, the PPEP program had visited over 80 secondary schools, mostly across South Australia but they can be contacted directly regarding plans to expand the program across other states.

New Zealand

Endometriosis New Zealand has a similar education program called ME (Menstrual Health and Endometriosis). This program has been running since 1995 and was included in a 2017 research study observing endometriosis education in schools and examining the impact of such an education program on early recognition of symptoms suggesting endometriosis. The study found strong suggestive evidence that consistent delivery of a menstrual health education program in schools increases adolescent student awareness of endometriosis. In addition, there is some evidence that in a geographical area of consistent delivery of the program, there was a shift in earlier presentation of young people assigned female at birth to a specialised health service.

United States

The creators of the documentary *Endo What?* have launched a school nurse initiative within the United States which aims to supply educational toolkits to school nurses, who are usually among the first to know when teenagers have endometriosis symptoms. The school kit includes a copy of their documentary which is suitable to show students, a poster to hang in the nurse's room, a downloadable discussion guide to promote open dialogue and communication between nurses, teachers, administrators and students, as well as a downloadable sample lesson plan for health teachers to teach a class about endometriosis.

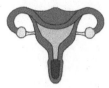

Finally, I want you to know that high school is not the be all, end all. I always want you to try your best and even if that isn't enough to get you where you want to be, there will be other ways. High school does not determine the course of your life and neither does your pain. Do what you can, and know that you still have so much ahead of you. You are more than your final score!

" It's not resting bitch face, it's just a bitch that needs rest. **"**

MIMI BUTLIN

13

Rest and play

Self-care

It is so crucial that we, as human beings, look after our mind, body and soul but I'll be the first to admit, it is so much easier said than done! I mean, look at us. We are living in a world that is rushed, demanding and ever-changing. Our work-life balance is in constant limbo and we are drowning in social feeds that are crying for affirmation and comparison. We often put others first, me-time is pretty low on the list of priorities and when we bump it up, we are ridden with guilt.

You and I both know that dealing with a condition like endometriosis comes with stress. From physical pain to mental and financial challenges as we try to deal with it all in the right way—it is exhausting! It also doesn't help that your endo symptoms worsen when you're under the pump from external sources like work or what is happening in the world (2020, anyone?). Because of this, you often feel like a burden on everyone and consequently, you fall into this mindset that your body is undeserving of love and self-care.

Self-worth is deeply affected by chronic illness and the neglect that comes with it. Think about it, if our human need to be cared for is rejected through attitudes of medical professionals and societal expectation, it has a knock-on effect on how we care for ourselves. This is something that I have definitely struggled with, but you know what? Enough is enough! It's time to snap out of this negative attitude towards ourselves and start attending to our needs. We NEED some self-care!

What is self-care?

By definition, self-care is the practice of taking action to preserve or improve one's own health.

It comes in all shapes and sizes because no two people are the same. What makes me feel good might be the complete opposite for you, and that's okay! Self-care can be as simple as taking the dog for a walk, switching on a mindfulness/meditation app or cooking a nice meal. Doing a jigsaw puzzle or reading a book. It's whatever YOU need to do to feel warm, fuzzy and in tune with your fine self.

What's more, self-care isn't just a one-time quick fix. It needs to be a continuous action and, like endo, it requires a whole-body approach. We're talking physical, mental, emotional, spiritual—all of it! Even the professional aspect of our lives deserves to be in on the action.

So, how do we do self-care? A good way to start is by taking a moment to stop and think about the times you have felt good and fulfilled. Where were you? What were you doing? Who were you with? Write all this down, pinpoint whether it was an object or an experience and figure out if it is something you can replicate as part of your shiny new self-care routine.

Second, schedule it into your life. Especially if you are a busy bee, put some self-care into your diary like it's an appointment and mark it as high importance (because it is!). The duration is entirely up to you. We all follow different routines so whether it's a five-minute or one-hour practice, it's whatever you can fit in that's going to improve your wellbeing.

Self-care doesn't have to be expensive either. In today's world, there are sooo many organisations and brands trying to capitalise on this concept and, in a sense, self-care has turned into its own marketplace. This can be good in that it can bring global recognition to a much-needed ritual, and it may also help you find new things that you love. On the other hand, commodification can be Kinda Gross and our needs shouldn't be taken advantage of or turned into a marketing tool. Such strategies can downplay the seriousness of self-care which, by the way, has been recognised by the National Health Service in the UK as a legitimate practice.

To help you get the ball rolling, I thought I would share some of my personal favourite acts of self-care.

Bath

I feel like there's a bit of an attitude that baths are for babies and showers are for adults but, honestly, screw the haters and get that tap running because bathing is one of the ultimate ways to relax!

Having a bath really forces you to slow down and literally immerse yourself in warmth. This is turn calms your mind, muscles and nerves. Not only that, it's like a giant liquid heat pack and we know the benefits of heat relief for endo flare-ups. Bathing is also great for a restful night's sleep as your body temperature goes up and your body then works extra hard to reduce it, making you sleepy.

For that extra oomph, you could throw in a nice bath bomb—but only if you can be bothered cleaning it up afterwards, especially if it's a colourful one. I personally keep things pretty simple in terms of my bath. I love chucking in some Epsom salts which help the body's natural detoxification process and soothe tired muscles. They're easy to find at a supermarket or chemist. I also add a few drops of clary sage essential oil because of its antispasmodic properties and, hey, a li'l aromatherapy never hurt nobody (except if you are pregnant: use essential oil with caution because some are not preg-friendly). Light some candles, chuck on some music, a podcast or even your fave TV show. No judgement here if you wanna get nostalgic with some bubble bath or toys too. You do you, boo.

Reality TV binge

Whether it's the sickening looks served on *RuPaul's Drag Race*, the drama of *Keeping up with the Kardashians* or the wholesome makeovers in *Queer Eye*, I have no shame in declaring my love for reality TV. It's an easy watch that serves as a welcoming escape and distraction from my pain and other stresses in my life.

Chocolate

Ah, yes, my one true medicine. Chocolate is like the definition of indulgence, right? There's this fancy organic fig and wild orange flavour you can find at the supermarket and health shops that is my ULTIMATE. What makes an orange wild, btw? I just visualise a cute little orange running freely in the forest, is that a wild orange? Anyway, this little block'o'choc is, like, $7 so I only get it when I really need it but, on the plus side, it's gluten and dairy free!

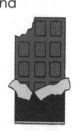

Massage and pedicure

These are things that I don't get very often but when they happen, it feels like a real treat. Reduced muscle tension and a pretty set of nails, I love this for me!

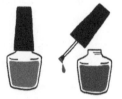

Red wine and a platter

There's no other reason than red being my drink of choice and platters make me feel fancy. Depending on your tolerances, this may be a recipe for a flare-up but sometimes you just gotta throw all f*cks out the window and go for it!

Face mask/sheet

While I am extremely pro-mask for the pandemic, I'm not referring to the ones we use for COVID-19. I'm talking about those cold, gooey sheets of goodness that scream PAMPER! and provide such a therapeutic sensation. They are hydrating, detoxifying and that fresh, airy feeling when you peel one off is SO satisfying. Face masks would

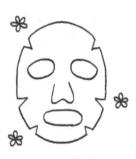

have to be one of the first things that spring to mind when you think of self-care and they're so easy to find. Have a suss online or check out the beauty section in your local supermarket, pharmacy or department store. Alternatively, you can buy face masks in the form of a cream and apply yourself.

Saying no

This one might sound a bit random because I feel like we are constantly told to say yes to people and opportunities. I mean, there's a whole film called *Yes Man*. But let's be realistic, you cannot and should not be expected to say yes to everything, especially when you are suffering.

We want to always show up for people, meet their expectations and make them happy, but as a chronic-illness sufferer, this can easily turn into a destructive habit that comes at a cost. Our health. When you don't honour yourself and your needs, you may start to foster resentment and regret. This can lead to even more self-critique and negative self-talk, which isn't fun.

Given the nature of my work in radio, a lot of people assume that I'm super extroverted but I'm really quite the opposite. My friends know me as a nanna and, sure, I've probably lost some because they think I'm not fun or social enough. However, that just means I get to invest more energy into the friends that respect and understand my boundaries and limitations as someone who works a demanding full-time job while dealing with endo. Saying no is never going to be easy, I know that. But sometimes for the sake of our health and wellbeing, we just have to do it.

Living with endometriosis means we tend to blame our bodies for a lot of things, but we need to start loving them.

We need to change the mindset that our body is working against us when it's actually trying to *protect* us from pain. We should be *rewarding* our bodies for looking out for us and self-care is a good way to do that.

So, repeat after me, self-care ISN'T selfish! It's an ongoing practice that is key in maintaining a healthy state of mind and preventing burnout.

As RuPaul says: 'If you can't love yourself, how in the hell you gonna love somebody else?'

AMEN!

Play

Hands up if you've ever made super fun plans for the weekend that you've been looking forward to *so much* only to spend it in bed with endo pain? I see you!

Throughout my mid- to late-twenties, I have found it harder and harder to keep up with my various friendship circles. I used to be somebody who could hit up three live music shows a week with ease but now I'd be lucky to come out of one without feeling completely exhausted. While my friends are searching for the closest bar within the venue, I'm looking around for a seat or a wall I can lean on. I'm usually the first to leave a night out and often pull a Houdini (or practise ghosting, as some call it) because I simply cannot be fucked explaining to my drunk buddies why I'm tired or in pain or that if I keep drinking my ovaries will be super pissed (pun always intended). Weekends away also require more planning than they used to in case a random flare-up appears out of nowhere. It can be a hard pill to swallow but the reality is that these days, my social life is less about spontaneity and more about preparation.

While there are going to be days when everything sucks and we feel left behind as the world keeps turning, endometriosis doesn't have to be a total life sentence! Easier said than done, I know. But we can still be social, we just have to be a bit more strategic about how we do it. So, let's suss our options!

When you do go out . . .

You will have your good days when you feel in control of your body and you deserve to celebrate these moments! If you head out somewhere, take a moment to plan ahead to save future you any potential distress. Pack some painkillers and stick-on heat pads, which I personally find sit really well on high-waisted underwear. If you're anticipating your period, wear some period undies. They don't feel any different to your usual knickers, but the built-in pad will have you covered in case there's any unexpected leakage.

Suss out the area and see whether it is close to public transport or if the parking is accessible. Even check if there are nearby pharmacies or medical centres should you need them. If it's a venue, google whether there's seating. To ease any potential anxiety, let a loved one know where you are going and ask if they could be on stand-by to pick you up should you suddenly feel any symptoms arise.

Track your pain

I've already mentioned the benefits of diarising your pain and symptoms throughout the book, and it can really come in handy when planning social events. For example, my period is (fortunately) very regular and because I know when it's coming, I will always avoid pencilling in a catch-up or anything that requires effort, really! Contrary to Bhad Bhabie, you can cash me *inside*.

Don't shame a stay-in

Speaking of! If you can't go out, it's not the end of the world. As a proud couch hermit and devoted dressing-gown wearer, I can absolutely vouch that staying in is COOL. It's cheap, it's comfortable and it can be social!

Case in point: sleepovers. Yep, I'm talking about the ones you did in primary school. The best part of growing up! I remember them so vividly—sleeping bags spread across the lounge room floor as my friends and I would guess what soft drink we were sipping on blindfolded, while *Crossroads* was playing in the background (#FreeBritney). Those were THE DAYS.

Chuck on a movie or TV series, get some board games, whip out some snacks or get food delivered and chill! I reckon this totally beats a lunch or dinner out because you don't have to dress up and you're not limited to a set menu. You can eat and drink whatever you feel like! You are spoiled for choice of screen entertainment thanks to all the streaming services and, hey, if you feel crappy, heat relief is only a few steps away in the form of microwaving a heat pack or plugging in your electric heat pad. Bonus points if you have a guest bedroom so you and your mates can avoid sleeping bags on the lounge room floor.

Or if a daytime catch-up is more your thing, invite someone over for a cup of tea or coffee (whatever you can stomach, really). This is a great alternative if you're not able to head out but still want to see your friends. I also think opting for a beverage as opposed to a sit-down meal creates less pressure in terms of the duration of your hangout.

All it takes is a text: 'I'm not feeling up to heading out but I would still love to see you, so you are welcome to pop over for a tea and we can catch up.'

Plus, if COVID-19 showed us anything, it is that despite being physically apart, you can still be social in isolation. From trivia zoom nights to facetiming over a meal or drink, the pandemic forced people to get creative with how they interact. One of my favourite hobbies that I picked up in lockdown was live streaming aerobics classes with a few of my colleagues. Not only was it a great way to stay connected, but we all got to try something new together and have a few laughs as we dressed in our finest eighties attire and grapevined into the weekend.

All of these things became part of the 'COVID-19 normal' and I'm super hopeful that it's helped our mates gain a better understanding of the times when our endo pain has not allowed us to leave the house.

Seeking extra support

I really rate support groups, especially the fact that they are not only *so* accessible but mostly free! It's really special to be able to connect with others who know exactly what you're going through, and this can be done in various formats. Online support groups are particularly great for those days when you just cannot leave the house and also for people living in rural and regional areas. Face-to-face support group gatherings will usually take place somewhere that's been decided by the group so that everyone's needs are met. Some organisations like QENDO host various meet-ups across Australia but, alternatively, you could always organise one in your area!

how to help

" Privilege is not something I take and which [I] therefore have the option of not taking. It is something that society gives me, and unless I change the institutions which give it to me, they will continue to give it, and I will continue to have it, however noble and equalitarian my intentions. **"**

HARRY BROD

14

Endo is for everyone

From the constant misunderstanding and dismissal of our pain to missing out on work and social occasions, endometriosis has long proven to be an isolating experience. I've descended to the very depths of loneliness with this condition, but I have also found great comfort within our patient community. Unfortunately, not everyone with endo can say the same.

Being a cisgender white woman, I am the billboard for a lot of things in life. I mean, you literally do hear me on the radio because that is my job, but I'm also what you see on TV and in magazines. I'm what you see in window displays and shopfronts, as well as the brochures and posters that greet you upon stepping inside a medical clinic. I am 'women's health'. I am endometriosis and what doctors and society view in terms of research and awareness. I think this needs to change.

Reading that might leave you a bit confused. *Bridget, what do you mean? Didn't it take years to receive your diagnosis? Didn't your financial situation prevent you from seeing a gynaecologist? Haven't medical professionals failed you?*

Yes, yes and yes. I have experienced hardships in life and most certainly throughout my endometriosis journey. We all have and I'm not here to discredit *any* of those challenges. What you and I have gone through is valid. But this book needs to be for *everyone* with endometriosis and if I am going to be a megaphone for endo, it's really important to me that everyone feels heard. That cannot be possible unless we give our black, Indigenous, people of colour (POC), queer, trans and gender-diverse mates the overdue recognition and inclusion that they deserve. Since basically forever, the conversations surrounding endo have been exclusive to cisgender white women and I believe it is on those of us who carry that privilege to help change this for the better.

To form a greater understanding of the issue at hand, let's start with dissecting what my privilege means. In her 2002 paper 'Understanding White Privilege', Frances E Kendall explains that white privilege is an institutional set of benefits granted to those of us who, racially, resemble the people who dominate the powerful positions in our institutions and establishments. One of the primary privileges is having greater access to power and resources than people of colour do; in other words, purely on the basis of our skin colour, doors are open to white people that are not open to other people. I'll give you an example. Those of us who are white can pretty much count on the fact that our nation's history books will be overwhelmingly white-centric. Whereas

Indigenous Australian, African American and Native American parents, for example, will know that their children are not as likely to learn in school about the contributions of their people. Growing up, my history curriculum mainly focused on white people. You know, English explorers like Matthew Flinders or John Edward Eyre. There was zero mention of Eddie Mabo, Woollarawarre Bennelong or any key Indigenous figure for that matter.

All of us who are white by race have white privileges, although the extent to which we have them varies depending on a few factors such as gender, sexuality, age, physical ability, socio-economic status etc. For example, looking at race and gender, we find that white men have greater access to power and resources than white women do. White men are paid more and they are pretty much the default for many medical research studies. Women have long faced greater disadvantages than men. But both genders can agree that because we are white, we know we are far less likely to be killed by the police. We know we are always going to see ourselves represented in the media. We know we are more likely to access better health care than black people. The world essentially revolves around whiteness ... and that ain't a good thing.

Now, we cannot change our privilege. You can't just opt out or unsubscribe. But we *can* change the system. And, honestly, we owe it to the entire human race to do so. Think about it. How bloody nice would it be to live in a world where everyone was equal? Where everyone with endometriosis could access the same care and resources? Where we all felt seen and supported? We have the power to make this happen but to get it done, we need to acknowledge where imbalance exists within the endometriosis community.

Race

Let's not beat around the bush here: gynaecology was *built* on racial injustice. Its history is long and deeply troubling.

James Marion Sims. Ever heard of him? Arguably the most famous American surgeon of the nineteenth century and the 'father of modern gynaecology', apparently. He developed pioneering tools and surgical techniques, but his practice was rooted in the slave trade, conducting gynaecologic research and non-consensual surgery on enslaved black women without anaesthesia in the 1840s. Why? According to historians, Sims believed that black women didn't experience pain the way white women did. Like, WTF?!

Fast-forward to the late 1930s and the assertion that endometriosis was linked to delayed pregnancy among white middle-class women. This conclusion was drawn by Boston gynaecologist Dr Joseph Meigs and it was based on his almost exclusively white clientele. A similar sentiment was echoed throughout the 1980s. As the documentary *Endo What?* reported, endometriosis was regarded as a 'career woman's disease' and was profiled around white, professional, highly educated women with insurance.

Even as recently as 2016, the Association of American Medical Colleges reported that half of white medical trainees believed African Americans had thicker skin or less sensitive nerve endings than white people. In 2018, an American study found that black patients were half as likely to be prescribed opioid drugs in emergency departments for non-definitive pain as opposed to white patients. Statistics from 2019 also show that black women were only about half as likely to be diagnosed with endometriosis compared with white women.

Racism has showed its ugly face throughout menstrual history too. Did you know that the sanitary belt was invented by Mary Beatrice Davidson Kenner? In 1956, Mary created an adjustable sanitary belt with a moisture-proof napkin pocket. This was long before the disposable sanitary pad, so menstruators relied on cloth and rags, but Mary's invention decreased the risk of blood leakages and stained clothes. It was a game changer! The following year, Mary was able to save up enough money to get her first patent which gave her a legal right to stop others from making or selling what she invented without permission. However, the first company that expressed interest in her creation, the Sonn-Nap-Pack Company, pulled out of the deal. Why? They discovered that Mary was African American. Mary never profited from the belt because her patent expired and became public domain, allowing it to be manufactured freely. Her invention was a revolutionary step for menstrual hygiene during a time when options were limited and often uncomfortable, yet she was never paid or credited for her pioneering work.

Have a think about how many public figures of colour are talking about endo. There are only a handful, like Whoopi Goldberg and American actress Tia Mowry. Everyone else is white. Mowry expressed concern about this in an interview with *Women's Health* magazine:

> *I thought I was alone because no-one I knew personally had dealt with this. And then I realised: I'd never really seen someone African American in the public eye talking about endometriosis or their struggles with infertility. And when you don't know or see anyone else who looks like you talking about what you're going through, you feel alone and suffer in silence.*

For this reason, Tia decided to continue speaking publicly about endometriosis and it even led her to releasing a cookbook, *Whole New You*, full of recipes for the diet she followed to decrease inflammation. She said:

I decided to put it all out there because I wanted to help people feel less alone—and supported. I also want to raise awareness. As black women, we're particularly at risk for endometriosis, yet so many of us don't even know what this condition is. If more of us talked about it, more women might say: 'Hey, I've had those symptoms, let me go get checked.' Compared to other communities, it feels like there's a void when it comes to talking about healthy living and medicine from African American women, for African American women.

Jenneh Rishe, co-founder of American non-for-profit organisation The Endometriosis Coalition, echoes this comment about representation.

I have found that, culturally, health is not something the African American community tends to speak about publicly in general. I had a difficult time getting this community to engage and found they were more comfortable messaging me privately. I found that there was a lot of misinformation circulating specifically within the African American community, and I think that can be attributed to not feeling comfortable reaching out to many of the other endo advocates and organisations that are predominantly white.

This issue is not limited to African Americans and, as we saw in 2020, the Black Lives Matter movement forced other countries to look at their own backyards. For us in Australia, that means reflecting on the barriers that our Indigenous communities face in particular. Did you know that Australian Indigenous women are 1.6 times less likely to be admitted to hospital for endometriosis? Various factors contribute to this statistic, such as difficulty accessing health care, the costs associated with treatment and cultural differences in healthcare-seeking behaviour. I remember speaking with one of my endogram followers who is Indigenous, and she said that while some of her relatives were suffering, conditions like endometriosis are simply not discussed in her mob. No-one is providing them with vital information or support and they are left to suffer in silence.

So, what needs to be done? For Jenneh Rishe, it starts with recognition.

I think acknowledging the negative history between the medical community and African American people is something that needs to be on the forefront of every healthcare practitioner's mind. There is a guard that is up and rightfully so. Learning cultural sensitivity and applying it to their practice has to be something they are constantly working towards.

Jenneh also outlines the need for a more welcoming and inclusive environment.

That could be as simple as sharing more black stories and black faces on our social media platforms or by addressing and educating about the inequities that black women face within healthcare.

The same goes within Australia. I would love to see the prevalence of endometriosis in our Indigenous communities become a real research priority, as well as funding for education programs in rural and remote areas. National organisations need to be leading the conversation and amplifying these voices and the medical community needs to look at providing culturally competent care so there is reduced inequality in healthcare outcomes. The 2018 National Action Plan for Endometriosis noted that there is a need for improved accessibility for people in rural and regional areas, as well as Aboriginal and Torres Strait Islander people, culturally and linguistically diverse communities, transgender and non-binary people, people with disabilities and disadvantaged groups. There was also a call for action in supporting the development of endometriosis-specific media and awareness materials that are tailored for these communities, however at the time of writing this book, I have not come across any public updates about actioning these points.

Gender and identity

I've had so many interactions with different people on endogram but one I will never forget was within the first few weeks of launching the account in 2019. I shared a post that read 'You Are Not Alone' with the caption highlighting stats on how many women suffer from endometriosis. I didn't think much of it, but that was the exact problem.

One person commented: 'Try to be aware not to use gendered language pls ... Non-binary, trans and other gender-diverse people are capable of getting endo (I myself am nb ... don't have endo but being nb (non-binary) makes me hyper aware of gendered language).'

You know how on the internet, people can be so quick to jump on things and shame others for getting something wrong, even if the intent was good? Especially without giving that person a chance to learn or even realise what they've done? It's partly why cancel culture is such a scary thing for people posting online. This person could have easily done that to me but, instead, they politely and fairly pointed out a big flaw in my attempts to raise awareness for endometriosis (Thank you Magnus!). I wasn't being inclusive and I really was coming from a position of privilege. I deserved to be held publicly accountable and I'm thankful that this follower did so in such a considered manner. Their comment really opened my eyes because, as a woman, I know firsthand how hard it has been for my pain and symptoms to be taken seriously. Can you imagine just how difficult it would be to navigate the medical system for a 'women's health' condition when you don't even identify with that gender?

A few months later, I shared a post to express how much I had learned regarding the use of gendered language within the endo community. The response was mostly positive, but one comment really irked me:

What offends me is y'all taking your eye off the ball. Bringing awareness and more research to a disease I've fought for 28 years. But sure, let's focus on this other thing ... cause we aren't taken ... seriously [enough] as it is. I'm not inclined to follow a page that cares more about the feelings of maybe .1% of your followers than the vast majority of your followers who have suffered with this wretched disease for decades. SJW (social justice warriors) everywhere.

Here's the thing, when we say that endo is for everyone, we are allowing more people to speak up, be heard and join the fight. The more the merrier! When we say that endometriosis is a 'women's health' issue, we are actively excluding and dismissing the experiences and struggles of those with endo who do not identify as female. Just ask Cori Smith from New York, a transgender man with endometriosis, who I had the pleasure of speaking to in September 2019 for *The Hook Up*, triple j's show on love and f*cking. No, really, that's the official program description. For Cori, the current language surrounding endo has had a huge effect. 'Honestly, it makes you feel unseen,' he told me. He went on:

It's very scary just being trans in the world today and then on top of that to find that the community that you thought would understand you the most, to be told that we're just a small percentage and that we don't matter so you shouldn't have to change your dialogue or language. It invalidates my entire lifelong battle with this disease, every surgery that I've had, all of the discrimination I've faced, not to mention the pain that I still experience today.

Someone else I spoke to for this package was Jess Tilley from my hometown of Ballarat. Jess identifies as non-binary and has been constantly misgendered throughout their consultations with various medical professionals.

Every time I saw a new doctor it was a whole new thing, like you just need to get pregnant and you just need to find the right boy, or you're a woman, why don't you do this? And it was really disheartening to hear that from people who are supposed to be professionals, that are supposed to help people no matter what.

Since our chat, I have been so proud to see Jess use their voice as a patient advocate and join QENDO as a facilitator for their inclusive Facebook support group, QENDO & Co.

To gain a professional perspective on endometriosis within the trans, gender-diverse and non-binary community, I reached out to Grace Lee. Grace is counsellor with Equinox, a trans and gender-diverse healthcare service in Melbourne. Established through extensive consultation with the trans, gender-diverse and non-binary (TGDNB) community, Equinox is a safe space where these patients can feel respected, understood and affirmed. Staff at Equinox include many TGDNB people and all staff have been trained in working with TGDNB patients, so they can explain processes in detail and can refer patients to TGDNB-affirmative specialist practices where needed.

Grace has witnessed firsthand the struggles that TGDNB patients face when it comes to seeking help for their health issues.

The medical system can be anxiety provoking and traumatic. Too often, the medical services make gendered assumptions about patients that just don't fit. Most endometriosis services will be categorised under gynaecology or women's health. This creates discomfort or distress for transmasculine people attending such services.

As Grace explains, negative experiences can start as early as booking an appointment. Having a masculine name and deeper voice can complicate things as clients may be questioned or asked to repeat their name or clarify if the appointment is for someone else. It can continue at reception and in the waiting area—again, patients may need to use their deadname from their Medicare card, and some practices insist on using that name for bookings, reports or prescriptions. This outs the patient again and causes anxiety and distress when they have to explain to reception or in front of other patients. Likewise, a patient might be called from the waiting room by a clinician using their deadname which will immediately out them to anyone else there.

Not to mention the medical procedures that involve intimate physical examinations. TGDNB patients may experience levels of gender dysphoria and dysmorphia that make such examinations extremely distressing and may result in them not presenting for examination. For those not sure of these terms, gender dysphoria involves a conflict between a person's sex assigned at birth and the gender with which they identify, and dysmorphia is where a person spends a lot of time worrying about flaws in their appearance.

According to Grace, a common experience in medical situations for TGDNB patients is that the clinician seeing them may not know or understand much about trans health. Grace says:

In these situations, the clinician often questions the patient as a way of educating themselves—placing a burden on the patient. Further, some clinicians will refuse to treat the patient because the clinician claims they don't understand the impacts of, for example, hormone therapies, and suggests that the patient see a specialist gender health practitioner. Many TGDNB patients will have experienced various forms of discrimination within health-service contexts and, coupled with past trauma, will often be anxious, hyper vigilant, and hypersensitive to the interaction with medical staff.

So, what can be done to ensure everyone with endo feels safe and included? For Grace, it's a joint effort between medical professionals and the patient community. Grace says:

Seeking education relating to trans-affirmative practices is critical. Patients should not be educating practitioners. It is important that practices review their procedures, their forms and record systems, their staff training and the principles on which they operate. Specialist training and capacity-building organisations are able to provide training, consulting and auditing across the range of services provided to TGDNB patients.

As for the wider patient community, it really starts with our own conversations. I recently attended a webinar on the role of Pelvic Therapy, hosted by Hela Health and Amy Stein. Not *once* in the hour-long session, did these two speakers mention the word 'women'. It was always about the patient. And it was so easy! When I talk about eliminating gendered language from our vocabulary, I don't mean that you cannot call ANYONE a woman ever again. You can always use your preferred personal pronouns when you are talking about yourself or if you're chatting to a group that you know all identify as women. That's fine and it makes sense! But when it comes to addressing large groups of people with endo, it's important to adjust our language to cater for that. It may seem a little difficult at first, but it will come naturally after some practice. A great starting point would be these examples adapted from The Endometriosis Network Canada.

INSTEAD OF ... ... TRY THIS

Instead of ...	... Try this
Hey ladies /girls /gals /guys !	Hey everyone/friends /fam/pals !
Women /girls with endometriosis	People with endometriosis
Endo sisters	Endo warriors Endoviduals Endo peeps Endo mates /friends /pals
1 in 10 women	1 in 10 people assigned female at birth

Adapted from The Endometriosis Network Canada

As Grace articulated so well, endometriosis is a condition that often results in patients suffering physical pain and mental distress. This is a shared experience that can bring patients together in supportive and helpful ways. Grace says:

Perhaps the endometriosis community can consider how it can provide support to all those who suffer with the condition. To acknowledge that this isn't simply the preserve of cis women, but that anyone who has or had a uterus (and those who never had one) are susceptible to this condition. For support groups and societies to think about how they present their services (often assuming those are exclusively for cis women), but rather to focus on the condition itself and the impact it has.

If you are trans, non-binary or gender diverse, you are valid. You deserve to be seen, heard and supported.

Alexa, play 'We're All in This Together' from *High School Musical.* ♡

"

Sometimes your friend circle decreases in size, but increases in value.

"

IVANA AND ANDREW VICK

15

For the friend, colleague, relative or partner

Hello loved one!

If you are reading this chapter, it's because someone who values you in their life wants you to know about something else that is a big part of their life—endometriosis. You may have witnessed their struggle at home firsthand or just noticed the suspiciously large number of heat packs lying around. Perhaps it was at work, with their empty desk greeting you more often than usual. Maybe you were sitting across from them at a lunchtime catch-up and spotted them squirming in their seat but insisting everything was fine. Perhaps you had no idea until now. Whether they passed this chapter on or you have sought out this book for your own learning, it means a lot that you are here.

Endometriosis can be a super hard thing to talk about for numerous reasons. I know I have struggled to explain my illness to others and quite often I will downplay it, simply because it is easier. It can be really exhausting telling people that it's actually so much more than a bad period and that it's not something that surgery, let alone yoga or celery juice, can 'fix'. When people with endo detail the true reality of their condition, they tend to feel like they are being a buzz-kill or they're worried that you'll think they're exaggerating because that's what some doctors have insisted. It can also feel like talking about their illness is accepting defeat; that they have lost control of it. But although they may struggle to find the words sometimes, they want you to know about their endo and how you can both deal with it to make your relationship the best it can possibly be. Your relationship deserves that.

By no means are you expected to be an expert on endo because honestly, this shit is complicated. But even just knowing the basics (see Chapter 1) and understanding the true meaning of chronic illness is a huge help.

When we talk about a chronic illness, we are talking about something that is long term and generally uncurable. Inconsistent in its pain and like a constant state of grey looming over our bodies, striking when it pleases. Sadly, chronic illness is remarkably common. In fact, nearly 50 per cent of Australians live with chronic illness—that's 11.4 million people. The reason it's perceived as rare, however, is because it is endured in secret. When you're fighting a battle that no-one can see, you have no choice but to adopt a strong poker face. In her recent interview with *Buzzfeed*'s deputy editor Lara Parker for *Vanity Fair*, writer Maham Hasan spoke about the complexities behind the term chronic illness:

> The word chronic, when you finally grasp it, is so hard to comprehend. It's like going through the death of a loved one because, over time, it gets a little easier to live with the fact, and then out of nowhere it will hit you really, really hard again.

Walking in our shoes

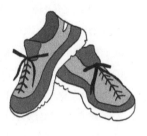

The COVID-19 pandemic drew some clear parallels to the chronic illness experience. Think about it: the unstable work, the sudden lack of physical inter-action and isolation. Heck, even panic buying, except we're talking stick-on heat pads rather than toilet paper.

The pandemic forced millions of people to confront a huge sense of uncertainty and the people who arguably endured it the best were those with chronic illness. Why? Because our lives didn't change *that* much. Don't get me wrong, the pandemic definitely presented problems for the chronically ill—surgeries were postponed and cancelled. Mine was in limbo but, luckily, I snagged a spot right in the tiny window of freedom before the second wave of COVID-19 hit Melbourne. There have also been limited appointments for physio and acupuncture, and even prescriptions for pain management have been affected. But a large portion of lockdown was already our reality.

Strangely, the one element of comfort from the global impact of COVID-19 was that it forced *everyone* to reassess how they live. We saw more effort and creativity in taking our social interactions online and overall a greater sense of empathy. Our loneliness was shared collectively and throughout the pandemic, you gained a taste of life with chronic illness. The one thing I would ask (and I say this with the biggest puppy eyes ever) is that you don't forget what you experienced—please, keep us in the picture.

Talk it out

For all relationships, whether they are intimate or professional, communication is key. But what should you say to something who is dealing with endometriosis? It can be an intimidating conversation for you to be part of, let alone initiate, so allow me to give you a heads up on some things we *really* appreciate hearing and things that should probs be avoided. Keep in mind, these are general tips and the choice of words should match your intimacy level.

☹ *What not to say* ☹

- ☛ *'Have you tried . . .'*
  On one hand, we know this is usually coming from a good place but before providing advice, especially if it is unsolicited, it would be really helpful to trust that we have spent *a lot* of time researching and trying anything and everything under the sun. Also consider whether your suggestion rides more on scientific backing or something like this . . .

- *'My friend's sister's cousin had endo but since having a kid/starting yoga, they're fine!'*

  It's important to remember how individualised endometriosis is and whilst it's super awesome that your friend's sister's cousin is feeling tops, that won't be the case for everyone. There is no known cause and no known cure for this condition and symptoms vary. Plus, it's very easy to interpret this kind of statement as a suggestion that we are not trying hard enough to help ourselves.

- *'Be positive.'*

  I'm all about optimism but telling someone to just be positive kinda implies that their symptoms or level of pain is dependent on their ability to be optimistic. If only it were that simple. Plus, a continuous emphasis on positive thinking is quite dismissive of chronic pain and leads to victim blaming. Positive thinking is literally not going to prevent the growth of my endo; it's not going to unstick my left ovary from adhesions. The reality is that people with good attitudes don't always overcome health problems and that is okay. It is okay to not be okay. Life isn't LEGO and in order to overcome any negative emotion, we have to acknowledge it's there. Toxic positivity does not allow that.

- *'But you don't look sick!'*

  Despite the fact that how I look is not always representative of how I feel, this statement implies we are lying about our illness, even though we have a medical diagnosis. Like, what do you need to see in order to believe me? The actual endo itself? I can scan you my surgery pics, will that do the trick? How do you want me to look?

🖤 *'You seemed fine yesterday!'*
It can be a damaging assumption that chronic illness means being bedridden 24/7 or that we cannot be 'fine' one day, and not the next. We're not faking being sick, we're faking being well.

😊 *What to say* 😊

🖤 *'I'm here to listen and support you.'*
This is a really nice and direct way of reassuring us that we are not alone and that we will be listened to without judgement.

🖤 *'How is your pain?'*
When asked how we are, we will usually say we're fine because it's easier. But by asking how our *pain* is, you are acknowledging that it's real.

🖤 *'What do you feel like eating. Let me drop something off for you.'*
Offering a specific item like food, or a particular gesture like helping with a chore, feels more effective than saying 'Let me know if you need anything' because it eliminates the pressure of us thinking of something that we need, which we might then think is too much of an imposition to ask for.

🖤 *'Don't sweat if you don't feel up for a catch-up/chat, I understand, and I'll be here when you're ready.'*

Trust me when I say that we feel like utter shit if we have to bail on plans. Saying something like this makes us feel less shit. There are going to be times when we can't see you or talk about what's going on, and there will be times when we may not want to. But please don't take our pain personally. It's not you and it's not us. It's endometriosis.

👉 *'I just wanted to check in and say that I'm thinking of you.'*
One of my oldest friends, Gemma, is the queen of sending these messages. We can go months without seeing each other but there's never any tension and she is always checking in on me. Such a simple gesture can bring so much comfort.

Your role

Endometriosis is a disease that sticks to our everyday decisions much like it attaches itself to our organs. It's persistent and exhausting. Its unpredictable nature can also cause significant changes to the dynamic of a relationship and the roles we play. For example, when Jenno and I started officially dating over four and a half years ago, never in our wildest dreams did we think that nights in with a heat pack would become the norm. Or that he would become the primary cook when I was in too much pain to function around the kitchen. At times, I have definitely felt more like a patient than a partner, but he always assures me that's not the case. And, let's be real, as long as the boy has his footy to watch or Tony Hawk's *Pro Skater 2* to play, he's chill.

If you know somebody with endo, anticipate that there will be shifts in your relationship. It's important to get on the same page and communicate any feelings or ideas concerning the responsibilities on both sides. We can't assume that everyone can read minds, so these conversations are super important to have.

I asked my endogram followers what else our loved ones can do to make life with endo just that little bit easier. They said:

- 'Pyjama parties and coming over to watch TV instead of going out.'
- 'Sit with me when it hurts too much to move.'
- 'Still invite us to things, even if we've said no before.'
- 'Understand that we are trying our best.'
- 'Accept our limitations.'
- 'Celebrate our good days and support our bad days.'

Look after yourself too

Have you ever heard of compassion fatigue? It's a legitimate condition that affects people who absorb the stress and emotions of those suffering from traumatic experiences like chronic or terminal illness. In order to treat these stresses, some good old self-care strategies need to be applied. It's a big red flag if you find yourself swirling helplessly in the chaos of chronic illness, unable to find your feet, so be sure to take time out for yourself and do what makes you feel good. We still want you to live a fulfilling life!

There are also support services that are available to you. I've seen numerous online groups for friends, family and partners of those with endo to connect and share tips with one another. Plus, the QENDO 24/7 support line is for anyone affected by endometriosis, PCOS and/or adenomyosis, and that includes carers, parents and partners. You can find the number at the end of this book alongside some other great resources you may want to check out.

Basically, don't set yourself on fire trying to keep others warm. You gotta look after yourself too.

"

Keep fucking fighting. **"**

HALSEY

A final word

So here we are . . . The end of the book! You made it! How are you feeling?

I hope you are feeling good. I hope you are feeling comfort in knowing that you are not alone and I hope that what you read in this book makes you feel empowered and better equipped in taking on your endometriosis on your own terms.

It's not easy, it never was, and you will still have your shitty moments. That's okay. But what I want you to know is that you can still live a beautiful life and you *deserve* to live a beautiful life, with or without endo.

It'll take some work; it'll take a few mistakes. There will be days where you feel like you are making progress only to stumble and fall but, my friend, you will get back up.

You will feel like you have lost part of yourself, but you will gain new parts that are wiser and stronger. Parts that don't take shit from nobody!

Life with endometriosis is not easy, but hopefully this book can help make it easier.

Now, go get 'em!

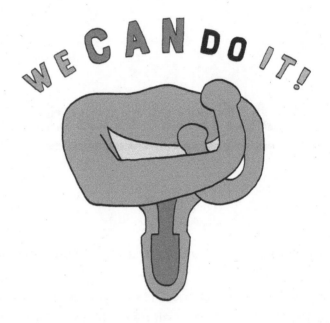

Acknowledgements

First, I would like to acknowledge the Wurundjeri people of the Kulin Nation who are the traditional custodians of the land which I have the absolute privilege to work and live on. I would also like to pay respect to the Wurundjeri Elders, past and present, and extend this respect to Aboriginal and Torres Strait Islander people from other communities who are reading this book.

Writing a book is never an easy feat but doing so in a unique time like 2020 was, uh, really something! Throughout the process of researching and drafting, I experienced two Melbourne lockdowns due to COVID-19, one endometriosis surgery, five painful periods and countless days of attempting to Get Shit Done on the couch, while my partner was shredding on guitar in his study, teaching students online. I was also working my regular full-time job so I might just quietly pat myself on the back.

However, *How to Endo* was not all me. This project has been a such a beautiful team effort and I simply could not have done it without the following people.

Claire Kingston, who believed I could use my voice through means of writing something so big like this. Tessa Feggans for helping me reach that glorious finish line and Alice Grundy and Emma Rafferty for making sure I did it in an articulate fashion. Words are hard! Alissa Dinallo for the fab cover design and Mika Tabata for the cute as heck illustrations; I'm particularly stoked we could get some nugs in here. My literary agent aka book wingwoman, Pippa Masson. Thank you all for answering my silly questions when I didn't know what the heck I was doing.

Every single legend who contributed to this book—Marika Day, Alison Harding, Lauren Gannon, Chantelle Otten, Jessica Taylor, Grace Lee, Jade Walker, Georgia Stuart, Claudia Wright, Brooklynn Chess, Jenneh Rishe, Elise Naismith, Katie Lovelock, Tori Hobbs and Swathi Sundaram. Thank you SO much for generously sharing your expertise and experiences.

To Mum and Dad, for your support and understanding as I went a little M.I.A. to get this done. I can't wait to come home again. To Jenno, for your never-ending patience despite always copping the full brunt of my stress and anxiety. I owe you a million VBs and potato cakes.

Shout-out to SBS Chill, ABC Classic and the Calming Acoustic playlist on Spotify. Your music proved to be very good background noise as I typed relentlessly on the couch. Highly recommend.

Iris Orbuch and Amy Stein, who I have never met but who educated me with their book, *Beating Endo*.

Last, but certainly not least—the endometriosis community. I am forever grateful for your support and I am constantly inspired by your passion and drive in raising awareness and advocating for better care. This is for you.

Recommended resources

Australia

QENDO—www.qendo.org.au
QENDO Helpline—1800 ASK QENDO (1800 275 73636)
Endometriosis Australia—www.endometriosisaustralia.org
EndoActive—www.endoactive.org.au
Pain Australia—www.painaustralia.org.au
Pelvic Pain Foundation of Australia—www.pelvicpain.org.au
Continence Foundation of Australia—https://www.continence.org.au/pages/how-
    do-pelvic-floor-muscles-help.html
Pain Link Helpline (call-back service)—1300 340 357

Worldwide

World Endometriosis Society—https://endometriosis.ca
Endometriosis.org—www.endometriosis.org
Nancy's Nook Endometriosis Education—https://nancysnookendo.com (or Nancy's
    Nook Endometriosis Education on Facebook)
Center for Endometriosis Care Patient Library—https://centerforendo.com/
    resources
International Pelvic Pain Society—https://www.pelvicpain.org
Endopaedia—www.endopaedia.info

Tame the Beast—www.tamethebeast.org (a free online education tool that aims to inspire research-based action in the treatment of chronic pain)

For support groups and organisations specific to your country, please visit http://endometriosis.org/support/support-groups/

Online tools

iCareBetter—https://endo.icarebetter.com

RANZCOG Rate Tool—https://ranzcog.edu.au/womens-health/patient-information-guides/other-useful-resources/rate

The Pain Perception Project—https://www.painperceptionproject.com

Books

Beating Endo—Iris Kerin Orbuch MD and Amy Stein DPT

Pain and Prejudice—Gabrielle Jackson

Documentary

Endo What?—www.endowhat.com

Endnotes

Chapter 1: Endo 101

p21   endometriosis classifications: Nikolaos Machairiotis et al., 'Extrapelvic endometriosis: a rare entity or an under diagnosed condition?', *Diagnostic pathology*, Vol 8(194), 2 December 2013, <www.ncbi.nlm.nih.gov/pmc/articles/PMC3942279/>

p21   varying appearances of endometriosis: Patrick Yeung Jr et al., 'Complete laparoscopic excision of endometriosis in teenagers: is postoperative hormonal suppression necessary?', *Fertility and Sterility*, Vol 95(6), 18 March 2011, pp. 1909–12, <www.fertstert.org/article/S0015-0282(11)00335-9/fulltext> and Dan Martin, *Laparoscopic Appearance of Endometriosis, Second Edition*, 1990–2020, Resurge Press, Richmond, accessed 2020, <www.danmartinmd.com/files/coloratlas1990.pdf>

p22   top twenty most painful health conditions: Gemma Mullin, 'NHS 20 most painful conditions', *The Sun*, 9 November 2019, <www.thesun.co.uk/news/10307035/nhs-reveals-20-most-painful-conditions/>

p24   'But this pain . . .': Gabrielle Jackson, *Pain and Prejudice*, Allen & Unwin, Crows Nest, 2019

p25   endometriosis theories and a number of factors: Center for Endometriosis Care, 'Endometriosis: A complex disease', 2018, accessed 2020, <www.centerforendo.com/endometriosis-understanding-a-complex-disease>

p25 one in nine have endo: Endometriosis Australia, 'Endo Facts', 2018, accessed 2020, <www.endometriosisaustralia.org/research>

p25 silent epidemic: Kathryn Perrott, 'Endometriosis: Health system "oblivious to suffering" of one in 10 women affected by "silent epidemic"', *ABC News*, 24 March 2017, <www.abc.net.au/news/2017-03-24/endometriosis-health-system-oblivious-to-suffering-of-women/8331534>

p25 it's not just a women's health issue: M. Zámečník and D. Hoštáková, 'Endometriosis in a mesothelial cyst of tunica vaginalis of the testis. Report of a case', *Cesk Patol*, Vol 49(3), June 2013, <www.ncbi.nlm.nih.gov/pubmed/23964911>

p26-7 fatigue: Endometriosis Foundation of America, 'Endometriosis Symptoms: Fatigue & Personality Changes', <www.endofound.org/fatigue-personality-changes>

p29 Endo has been classified into four stages: Neil P Johnson and Lone Hummelshoj et al., 'World Endometriosis Society consensus on the classification of endometriosis', *Human Reproduction*, Vol 32(2), 1 February 2017, <https://academic.oup.com/humrep/article/32/2/315/2631390>

p29 $837,433 to endometriosis research: Kathryn Perrott, op cit.

p30 evaluate physical attractiveness in women: P Vercellini and L Buggio et al., 'Attractiveness of women with rectovaginal endometriosis: a case-control study', *Fertil Steril.*, Vol 99(1), 2013, <https://pubmed.ncbi.nlm.nih.gov/22985951/>

p30 'We are way behind': Peter Rodgers, 'Priorities for Endometriosis', Research presentation, RANZCOG Annual Scientific Meeting 2019, <www.instagram.com/s/aGlnaGxpZ2hOOjE4MDc4MjYzOTU5MTg2MTkx?igshid=1muudgg45krng&story_media_id=2154837118852164473>

p30 National Action Plan for Endometriosis: Department of Health, Australian Government, July 2018, accessed 2020, <www.health.gov.au/resources/publications/national-action-plan-for-endometriosis>

p31 Hysterectomy does not cure endo: 'Ten Endometriosis Facts', *Endometriosis Australia*, 2014, accessed 2020, <www.endometriosisaustralia.org/endometriosis-facts>

p31 Pregnancy does not cure endo: Matthew Roser, 'Top 10 BS Myths About Endo', *Endo What?*, 16 June 2016, <www.endowhat.com/top-10-bs-myths-about-endometriosis/>

p32 Teenagers can get endo: Ros Wood et al., 'Myths and misconceptions in endometriosis,' *Endometriosis.org*, 20 November 2016, accessed 2020, <http://endometriosis.org/resources/articles/myths/>

p32 human foetus: C Bobel and I Winkler et al., 'The Womb Wanders Not: Enhancing Endometriosis Education in a Culture of Menstrual Misinformation', Palgrave Macmillan, Singapore, July 2020, < https://link.springer.com/chapter/10.1007/978-981-15-0614-7_22>

p32 Menopause does not stop endo: @endogirlsblog, Instagram, 22 July 2020, < www.instagram.com/p/CC6odygDund/?utm_source=ig_web_copy_link>

p32	Birth control does not stop endo: Ros Wood et al., op cit.
p33	Endometriosis is not a menstrual disease: @endogirlsblog, Instagram, 19 August 2020, <www.instagram.com/p/CECW3HYDX6u/?utm_source=ig_web_copy_link>
p33	Endometriosis is not the endometrium: Ros Wood et al., op cit.

Chapter 2: Diagnosis

p35	six and a half years for diagnosis: Endometriosis Australia, 'Endo Facts', 2020, <endometriosisaustralia.org/research>
p36	normalisation of period pain: G Hudelist and N Fritzer et al., 'Diagnostic delay for endometriosis in Austria and Germany: causes and possible consequences', *Human Reproduction*, Vol 27(12), December 2012, <https://academic.oup.com/humrep/article/27/12/3412/650946>
p36	Isaac Brown Baker: 'On the Curability of Certain Forms of Insanity, Epilepsy, Catalepsy, and Hysteria in Females,' *Manhattan College Omeka*, 1866, accessed 2020, <https://omeka-pilot.manhattan.edu/items/show/396>
p37	reddit thread: *Reddit*, June 2020, <www.reddit.com/r/Endo/comments/gutwl5/in_an_ask_reddit_thread_about_surprising/>
p40	RANZCOG/AGES guidelines for performing gynaecological endoscopic procedures: *RANZCOG*, first published 1993, last updated July 2019, <https://ranzcog.edu.au/RANZCOG_SITE/media/RANZCOG-MEDIA/Women%27s%20Health/Statement%20and%20guidelines/Clinical%20-%20Training/Guidelines-for-performing-gynaecological-endoscopic-procedures-(C-Trg-2).pdf?ext=.pdf>

Chapter 3: Surgery and recovery

p53	Orbuch recalls one patient . . . : Dr Iris Orbuch and Dr Amy Stein, *Beating Endo*, HarperCollins, New York, 2019, p. 213
p55	the splinter analogy: Dr Abhishek Mangeshikar, *The Indian Centre for Endometriosis*, Facebook, 13 July 2020, <www.facebook.com/endometriosisICE/posts/1003259433515672?comment_id=1004272660081016&reply_comment_id=1004398616735087>
p65	'this disease is by far': Dr Jeff Arrington, The Center for Endometriosis Care , Instagram, 8 May 2020, <www.instagram.com/p/B_7QiYpgWpt/?igshid=n79nrhb4jxrp&fbclid=IwAR2cKmINI44DiRSviiFlPcp6cvulLPtiMQcxEx7fXCNOcAq09HOTPJZwYHk>

Chapter 4: Associated conditions

p69	types of adenomyosis: Mohamed A Bedaiwy and Tommaso Falcone, 'Chapter 13—Endometriosis and Adenomyosis', *General Gynaecology*, 2007, pp. 321–45, <https://doi.org/10.1016/B978-032303247-6.10013-9>
p70	another key sign of adeno: G Levy and A Dehaene et al., 'An update on adenomyosis', *Diagnostic and interventional imaging*, January 2013, Vol 94(1), pp. 3–25, <https://pubmed.ncbi.nlm.nih.gov/23246186/>
p73	Rotterdam Criteria: Majid Bani Mohammad and Abbas Majdi Seghinsara, 'Polycystic Ovary Syndrome (PCOS), Diagnostic Criteria,

and AMH', *Asian Pacific Journal of Cancer Prevention*, 1 January 2017, Vol 18(1), pp. 17–21, <www.ncbi.nlm.nih.gov/pmc/articles/PMC5563096/>

p75   research suggests the nervous system is involved: Isabelle Amigues, 'Fibromyalgia', *American College of Rheumatology*, March 2019, <www.rheumatology.org/I-Am-A/Patient-Caregiver/Diseases-Conditions/Fibromyalgia>

p75–6   the severity and debilitating nature of some of the symptoms: B Walitt and RL Nahin et al., 'The Prevalence and Characteristics of Fibromyalgia in the 2012 National Health Interview Survey', *Plos One*, 17 September 2015, <www.ncbi.nlm.nih.gov/pmc/articles/PMC4575027/>

Chapter 5: Social media and self-advocacy

p84   approximately 70,000 health-related searches every minute: Margi Murphy, 'Dr Google Will See You Now: Search giant wants to cash in on your medical queries', *The Telegraph*, 10 March 2019, <www.telegraph.co.uk/technology/2019/03/10/google-sifting-one-billion-health-questions-day/>

Chapter 6: Let's get physical (therapy)

p99 $30,000 per year: Mike Armour et al., 'The cost of illness and economic burden of endometriosis and chronic pelvic pain in Australia: A national online survey', *Plos One*, 10 October 2019, <https://journals.plos.org/plosone/article?id=10.1371/journal.pone.0223316>

p110–11   Easy stretches to relax the pelvis: The Pelvic Pain Foundation of Australia, accessed 2020, <www.pelvicpain.org.au/easy-stretches-to-relax-the-pelvis-women/?v=ef10366317f4>

p113   the effect of yoga on the vagus nerve: Dr Iris Orbuch and Dr Amy Stein, *Beating Endo*, HarperCollins, New York, 2019, pp. 201–2

p114   in 2017, Brazilian researchers: Andrea Vasconcelos Gonçalves et al., 'The Practice of Hatha Yoga for the Treatment of Pain Associated with Endometriosis', *The Journal of Alternative and Complementary Medicine*, 1 January 2017, pp. 45–52, <www.liebertpub.com/doi/10.1089/acm.2015.0343>

Chapter 7: Mental health matters

p118   nearly 50 per cent stated they have experienced suicidal thoughts: Endometriosis UK, 'BBC research announced today is a wake-up call to provide better care for the 1.5 million people with endometriosis', 7 October 2019, <www.endometriosis-uk.org/news/bbc-research-announced-today-wake-call-provide-better-care-15-million-endometriosis-37606#.XyC5Jy1L3uO>

p127   1449 studies on mindfulness: 'The Honest Truth About Mindfulness', *Smiling Mind*, 14 May 2020, <https://blog.smilingmind.com.au/the-honest-truth-about-mindfulness-setting-yourself-up-for-success>

p128   as outlined by the MiCBT Institute: 'What is Mindfulness-integrated Cognitive Behaviour Therapy?', *MiCBT Institute*, accessed 2020, <https://mindfulness.net.au/what-is-micbt.html>

Chapter 10: Complementary therapies

p154   Dr Mike Armour for Endometriosis Australia: 'What Role Can Complementary Medicine Play In Managing Endometriosis', *Endometriosis Australia*, 2019, < www.endometriosisaustralia.org/post/2019/10/09/what-role-can-complementary-medicine-play-in-managing-endometriosis>

p156   TCM and the connection between mind, body and environment: K Rubi-Klein et al., 'Is acupuncture in addition to conventional medicine effective as pain treatment for endometriosis? A randomised controlled cross-over trial', *Eur J Obstet Gynecol Reprod Biol*, 2010, Vol 153(1), pp. 90–3, <https://pubmed.ncbi.nlm.nih.gov/20728977/>

p162   Look around your home . . . : Mary Ballweg, 'Endometriosis & dioxins: information for physicians, nurses, and other healthcare professionals', *Endometriosis Association*, January 1998, <www.researchgate.net/publication/272349987_Endometriosis_dioxins_information_for_physicians_nurses_and_other_healthcare_professionals_from_Endometriosis_Association>

p173   What's it got to do with endo?: 'Medicinal cannabis products: Patient information', Australian Government Department of Health: Therapeutic Goods Administration, 29 May 2018, <www.tga.gov.au/community-qa/medicinal-cannabis-products-patient-information>

p173   Persian texts: Natasha R Ryz et al., 'Cannabis Roots: A Traditional Therapy with Future Potential for Treating Inflammation and Pain', *Cannabis Cannabinoid Research*, Vol 2(1), 1 August 2017, pp. 210–16, <www.ncbi.nlm.nih.gov/pmc/articles/PMC5628559/>

p173   Queen Victoria's reign: J Russell Reynolds, 'On the therapeutical issues and toxic effects of cannabis indica', *The Lancet*, 22 March 1890, Vol 135(3473), pp. 637–8, <www.thelancet.com/journals/lancet/article/PIIS0140-6736(02)18723-X/fulltext>

p174   Georgia's positive experience echoes: Brian Mastroianni, 'Why do most patients use medical marijuana? Chronic pain', *Healthline*, 21 February 2019, <www.healthline.com/health-news/what-drives-patients-to-use-medical-marijuana-chronic-pain#The-results>

p174   a 2017 survey conducted by the NICM: Justin Sinclair and Dr Mike Armour, '1 in 10 women with endometriosis report using cannabis to ease their pain', *Western Sydney University*, 12 November 2019, <www.westernsydney.edu.au/newscentre/news_centre/more_news_stories/1_in_10_women_with_endometriosis_report_using_cannabis_to_ease_their_pain>

p175   Dr Mike Armour told *triple j Hack*: 'Apply Heat, Get High: This is how other women are dealing with endometriosis', *triple j Hack*, 3 October 2018, <www.abc.net.au/triplej/programs/hack/survey-looks-at-how-women-are-dealing-with-endometriosis-pain/10333996>

p175   How do I get it: 'Cannabis-based medicinal products', *National Institute for Health and Care Excellence*, 11 November 2019, <www.nice.org.uk/guidance/ng144/chapter/Recommendations#chronic-pain>

p176   the cost of medicinal cannabis alongside other barriers: Sophie Kesteven and Michele Weekes, 'Medicinal cannabis is legal in Australia, but people like Grace are still turning to the black market', *ABC News*, 2 July 2020, <www.abc.net.au/news/2020-07-02/medicinal-cannabis-use-in-australia-black-market/12387408>

Chapter 11: Fertility and parenting

p182   fertility is a tough conversation: Anusch Yazdani, 'Fertility and Endometriosis, should I worry?', *Endometriosis Australia*, accessed 2020, <www.endometriosisaustralia.org/post/2016/12/05/fertility-and-endometriosis-should-i-worry>

p183   infertility definitions: WHO-ICMART, <www.who.int/reproductivehealth/topics/infertility/definitions/en/>

p184   'I found it peculiar that my future . . .': Zara McDonald, *The Space Between*, Penguin Random House Australia, Sydney, 2020

p185   Acupuncture is worth a shot too: Caroline A Smith et al., 'Acupuncture performed around the time of embryo transfer: a systematic review and meta-analysis', *Biomed Online*, March 2019, Vol 38(3), pp. 364–79, <https://pubmed.ncbi.nlm.nih.gov/30658892/>

Chapter 12: Work and study

p201   American actress Mae Whitman: Jenny McCoy, 'Mae Whitman: "Endometriosis Is Like Being Shot With a Cannonball in the Stomach"', *Glamour Magazine*, 21 May 2020, <www.glamour.com/story/mae-whitman-on-navigating-a-hollywood-career-while-battling-endometriosis>

p202   'If you come to work with a flu': Jacinta Parsons, 'Pandemic has highlighted just how fragile we always were', *The Sydney Morning Herald*, 29 September 2020, <www.smh.com.au/lifestyle/health-and-wellness/pandemic-has-highlighted-just-how-fragile-we-always-were-20200929-p5609d.html>

p203   sick leave: Shalailah Medhora, 'Endometriosis costs the economy up to $7.4 billion a year in lost productivity, research finds', *triple j Hack*, 5 June 2019, <www.abc.net.au/triplej/programs/hack/endometriosis-endo-costs-economy-in-lost-producitivity/11183166>

p206   supporting workers with endometriosis in the workplace: Safe Work Australia, <www.safeworkaustralia.gov.au/doc/supporting-workers-endometriosis-workplace>

p206   Endometriosis Friendly Employer scheme: Endometriosis UK, <www.endometriosis-uk.org/endometriosis-friendly-employer-scheme>

p215   School programs: Deborah Bush et al., 'Endometriosis education in schools', *ANZJOG*, 28 March 2017, Vol 57(4), <https://obgyn.onlinelibrary.wiley.com/doi/abs/10.1111/ajo.12614>

Chapter 13: Rest and play

p 221   self-care as legitimate practice: Dr Bruce Warner, 'What does "self-care" mean and how can it help?', *NHS*, 17 November 2017,

Chapter 14: Endo is for everyone

p 232   a greater understanding of the issue: Frances E Kendall, 'Understanding White Privilege', 2002, <www.cpt.org/files/Undoing%20Racism%20 -%20Understanding%20White%20Privilege%20-%20Kendall.pdf>

p 234   James Marion Sims: Brynn Holland, 'The "Father of Modern Gynecology" Performed Shocking Experiments on Slaves', *History*, 29 August 2017, <www.history.com/news/the-father-of-modern-gynecology-performed-shocking-experiments-on-slaves>

p 234   endometriosis was linked to delayed pregnancy among white middle-class women: 'An Open Letter to the endometriosis community', Center for Endometriosis Care, 2020, <http://centerforendo.com/openletter>

p 234   Association of American Medical Colleges reported: Janice A. Sabin, 'How we fail black patients in pain', *Association of American Medical Colleges*, 6 January 2020, <www.aamc.org/news-insights/how-we-fail-black-patients-pain>

p 234   in 2018, an American study: Astha Singhal et al., 'Racial-Ethnic Disparities in Opioid Prescriptions at Emergency Department Visits for Conditions Commonly Associated with Prescription Drug Abuse', *Plos One*, Vol 11(8), 8 August 2016, <www.ncbi.nlm.nih.gov/pmc/articles/ PMC4976905/>

p 234   black women were only about half as likely to be diagnosed: Bob Kronemyer, 'How race/ethnicity influences endometriosis', *Contemporary OBGYN*, 23 May 2019, <www.contemporaryobgyn.net/ view/how-raceethnicity-influences-endometriosis>

p 235   racism has shown its ugly face throughout menstrual history: Zing Tsjeng, 'The Forgotten Black Woman Inventor Who Revolutionized Menstrual Pads', *VICE*, 9 March 2018, <www.vice.com/en_us/article/mb5yap/ mary-beatrice-davidson-kenner-sanitary-belt?fbclid=IwAR3x1M_A-sasjlXjIlhq36PCOHaL42OgpvXQfdz-yeS5CfLva590ilYVyq4>

p 235   how many public figures of colour are talking about endo: Tia Mowry 'My Extreme Pelvic Pain Turned Out To Be Endometriosis', *Women's Health Magazine*, 29 October 2018, <www.womenshealthmag.com/ life/a24400329/tia-mowry-endometriosis-black-women/>

p 237   this issue is not limited to African Americans: Australian Institute of Health and Welfare, 'Endometriosis in Australia: prevalence and hospitalisations', Canberra, 2019, <www.aihw.gov.au/getmedia/ a4ba101d-cd6d-4567-a44f-f825047187b8/aihw-phe-247.pdf. aspx?inline=true>

p 238   National Action Plan for Endometriosis: Department of Health, Australian Government, July 2018, accessed 2020, <www.health.gov. au/resources/publications/national-action-plan-for-endometriosis>

p 240   Cori Smith from New York: Bridget Hustwaite, Cori Smith and Jessica Tilley, 'Navigating reproductive health when you're trans', *The Hook Up Podcast (triple j)*, 30 September 2019, <www.abc.net.au/radio/programs/the-hook-up-podcast/navigating-reproductive-health-when-youre-trans/11561914>

p 244   examples adapted from The Endometriosis Network Canada: 'It's Time for the Endometriosis Community to Drop Gendered Language', *The Endometriosis Network Canada*, 25 June 2020, <https://endometriosisnetwork.com/blog/its-time-for-the-endometriosis-community-to-drop-gendered-language>

Chapter 15: For the friend, colleague, relative or partner

p 248   nearly 50 per cent: Tracey Bowden and Amy Donaldson, 'Nearly 50 per cent of Australians now have a chronic disease—many of them preventable', *ABC News*, 1 July 2019, <www.abc.net.au/news/2019-07-01/fifty-percent-of-australians-have-chronic-disease-health/11227298>

p 249   the word chronic: Maham Hasan, 'A BuzzFeed Editor's New Book Takes on a Once-Taboo World of Chronic Pain', *Vanity Fair*, 6 October 2020, <www.vanityfair.com/style/2020/10/a-buzzfeed-editors-new-book-takes-on-a-once-taboo-world-of-chronic-pain>

Full-page quotes

pxii   'Tell the story of the mountains . . .': Morgan Harper Nichols, Instagram, 2019 <www.instagram.com/p/Bw2dsqRgFae/?utm_source=ig_web_copy_link>

p 34   'It is imperative to look beyond gendered health . . .': Center for Endometriosis Care, 'Endometriosis: A complex disease', 2018, accessed 2020, <www.centerforendo.com/endometriosis-understanding-a-complex-disease>

p 50   'They now have chewable Viagra . . .': Amy Schumer, Oprah's 2020 Vision Tour Visionaries, *YouTube*, 18 January 2020, <www.youtube.com/watch?v=BodCxVdpYjY>

p 66   'You are never alone in this experience . . .': Stephanie Chinn, Instagram, 2020, <www.instagram.com/p/B--DHBIFyeT/?utm_source=ig_web_copy_link >

p 116   'One of the most difficult factors of this . . .': Jenny McCoy, 'Mae Whitman: "Endometriosis Is Like Being Shot with a Cannonball in the Stomach"', *Glamour Magazine*, 21 May 2020, <www.glamour.com/story/mae-whitman-on-navigating-a-hollywood-career-while-battling-endometriosis>

p 130   'I don't know who needs to hear this . . .': Lara Parker, Twitter, 26 August 2019, <https://twitter.com/laraeparker/status/1165678516911796224?s=20>

p 180   'You don't have to give birth to have a family': Jessica Murnane, Instagram, 21 August 2020, <www.instagram.com/p/CEHOQBujozc/?utm_source=ig_web_copy_link>

p 218   'It's not resting bitch face, it's just a bitch that needs rest': Mimi Butlin, Instagram, 2019, <www.instagram.com/p/B1Z0zfkAcQm/?utm_source=ig_web_copy_link>

p230   'Privilege is not something I take': Harry Brod in Michael S Kimmel and Michael Messner (eds), 'Work Clothes and Leisure Suits: The Class Basis and Bias of the Men's Movement', *Men's Lives*, Macmillan, New York, 1989, p. 280

p 246   'Sometimes your friend circle decreases . . .': Ivana and Andrew Vick, Instagram, 16 October 2020, <www.instagram.com/p/CGYAgT9jjOj/?utm_source=ig_web_copy_link>

p 256   'Keep fucking fighting': Halsey, 'Halsey's Tearful Acceptance Speech from the 2018 Blossom Ball', *Endometriosis Foundation of America*, 20 March 2018, <https://www.endofound.org/watch-and-read-halseys-tearful-acceptance-speech-from-the-2018-blossom-ball>

Index